A TRIAL OF
HORATIO'S STORY

Meg Harris Williams   *Photo: Adrian Williams*

By the same author:

Inspiration in Milton and Keats
A Strange Way of Killing: The Poetic Structure of Wuthering Heights
The Apprehension of Beauty (with Donald Meltzer)
The Chamber of Maiden Thought: Literary Origins of the
    Psychoanalytic Model of the Mind (with Margot Waddell)

for children:

Five Tales from Shakespeare

THE ROLAND HARRIS TRUST LIBRARY

A TRIAL OF FAITH:
HORATIO'S STORY
Hamlet in Analysis

Meg Harris Williams

The Clunie Press

London
KARNAC BOOKS

First published in 1997 by
H. Karnac (Books) Ltd.
58 Gloucester Road
London SW7 4QY

British Library Cataloguing in Publication Data

A C.I.P. record for this book is available from the British Library

ISBN 1 85575 127 2

Edited, designed, and produced by Communication Crafts

10 9 8 7 6 5 4 3 2 1

ACKNOWLEDGEMENTS

This story of an adolescent breakdown is based faithfully on the aesthetic and emotional structure of Shakespeare's *Hamlet*, and has been supervised throughout from the psychoanalytic point of view by Dr Donald Meltzer.

OPHELIA: O, what a noble mind is here o'erthrown!
The courtier's, soldier's, scholar's, eye, tongue, sword,
Th'expectancy and rose of the fair state,
The glass of fashion and the mould of form,
Th'observed of all observers, quite, quite down!

[III. i. 152–156]

CAST OF CHARACTERS

Dr David Horacio—a psychoanalyst
Antigone and Ismene Horacio—his daughters

Claude Dane—a wealthy industrialist
Gertrude Dane—his wife
Hamlet Dane—an English student at Cambridge University

Professor Antony Polack—a professor of English at
      Cambridge University
Ophelia Polack—a music student at Cambridge University
Nando Polack—her brother

Mrs Forte—a journalist
Forte—her son

Rosenfeld and Gildstein—students, friends of Hamlet

CONTENTS

CHAPTER EIGHT

The King and Queen

Breaching his own analytic technique, Horacio dines with Hamlet's parents and discovers something rotten in the state of Denmark which mirrors personal problems of his own. His first suspicions that these might have interfered with his relationship with Hamlet.

CHAPTER NINE

Ophelia at Colonus

Again against his professional judgement, Horacio agrees to a consultation with Ophelia. This confirms the disturbing effect of her beauty on Hamlet, but also makes clear Hamlet's ignorance of her character. Still Horacio has not fathomed the completeness of his own mistake.

CHAPTER TEN

Bottom's Dream

Horacio is bitterly disappointed by Hamlet on his return eight years later, after having followed the "Forte" road to intellectual yuppydom. Bottom's Dream explains Hamlet's flight years before, but only now does Horacio begin to understand his own mismanagement of the analysis.

CHAPTER ELEVEN

Horacio Agonistes

Finally this becomes clear during his own dream of Gertrude and of Ophelia, pulling together strands from his personal life and from Hamlet's analysis. Accepting their mutual interference at last, the "old romantic" is ready to review his own story.

A TRIAL OF FAITH: HORATIO'S STORY

The Prelude

O God, Horatio, what a wounded name
Things standing thus unknown, shall I leave behind me.
If thou didst ever hold me in thy heart,
Absent thee from felicity awhile,
And in this harsh world draw thy breath in pain
To tell my story.

[V. ii. 349–354]

November 1981

That interesting book by the melancholy young Dane with its grindingly repetitive yet fascinating spirals of sentences lay open where I had left it that Sunday afternoon before taking the dog for his afternoon walk. The small circular table near the window was where I preferred to sit and read. Now it was dusk, and it was my custom always to draw the curtains as my narrow, terraced house in Flask Walk, which also contained my consulting-room, exposed me to the view of passing patients—many of whom lived locally. As I moved past the table, I clumsily jogged my right arm, which was in plaster owing to an absurd accident I had had the previous night and surprisingly painful. The light from the two tall Georgian windows leapt over the basement chasm and glistened on the wet, narrow, uneven pavement outside (characteristic of the old village of Hampstead). It reached to the place where tree roots pushed the stone upwards. A young woman wearing large training shoes strode through the light squares as I closed the curtain, going in the direction of the village. There was a temporary lull in the rainy stormy weather, which had been blustering on for the past fortnight, though at the end of the road in the darkness where the massed trees and wide spaces of the Heath began, the energies of the storm still growled with the soughing of branches in the wind.

Since living alone I had become a voracious reader. I imagined Kierkegaard, who had compared himself with Shakespeare's Hamlet, stalking the flat pavements of Copenhagen, pursuing his compulsive strategy of spying on Regine (his Ophelia) in order to wean himself away. (Elsinore too was flat—its cliffs and abysses, drawing into madness, belonged to the topography of the mind, not the earth.) "If I had had faith, I would have stayed with Regine." What a brilliant insight! This was the phrase, in translation of course, which had been revolving in my own mind that afternoon as I walked with the dog in the chill soggy air, warming me from within like a glass of claret. And yet, to the casual reader—to one whose hunger for a certain truth had not sharpened his appetite to seize on such a phrase as eager prey—it might (like the "Beauty is Truth" of Keats's Grecian Urn) seem a trite commonplace devoid of meaning, a romantic excuse, a capitulation to social acceptability. "Marriage is good for you."

> In this harsh world draw thy breath in pain
> To tell my story.

>   [V. ii. 353–354]

Those words, too. It was now eight years since I had had my Hamlet in analysis, though less than a week since I had seen him last. In those eight years, society had changed, my personal life had changed, the world had changed, Hamlet had changed from the surly, rebellious young prince who had first enthralled me and become a pillar of the establishment—not actually a psychoanalyst, but what was bad enough, an omnipotent social analyst. This was a route that doubtless satisfied any craving he had for apostolic functioning, without being overtly directed against me. But why had he felt the need to take that road at all? Why the urgency, why the weakness? What had happened since that brief but intense period of analysis he had had with me? Broken off prematurely after less than a year, it had lain suspended cocoon-like in my memory, serving (I had always assumed) through the small amount of good we had achieved to keep his insight alive until the moment when he realized he would need to resume.

My dog, a huge and elderly Pyrenean mountain dog with long white hair, thumped his tail as he lay down on the Chinese rug and scattered some damp leaves over the beautifully waxed, wide wooden floorboards of my small and elegant sitting-room. I had a vivid memory of how ten or twelve years ago, in what seemed like another existence, those boards had been covered with a cheap rubber-backed carpet to absorb the noise of the clatterings and shrill clamourings of our two little girls, modulated by the regular admonitions of Beatrice: "Be quiet! Daddy's working, down below." A ghost in the cellarage, my consulting-room being directly underneath. How very different were my anxieties about work interference now! How different my worry about my daughters! (I was still fulminating over events in the restaurant last night, more in anger than in depression). And how was it that what had once been a joyful love affair with psychoanalysis now seemed to have become an enslavement ("workaholism", my daughter called it)? Then, for eight years, I had been waiting . . . for what? for Hamlet's return—for the resumption of our work, which I now saw could never be? The waste, the futility! But why should the history of Hamlet and his family and friends have affected me so deeply? Feelings and associations had been stirred up during the past week which clustered around this aborted analysis in such a way that it seemed to be coming to represent the focus of my discontent with my life, even the source of my anger with my own family. Was Hamlet a personification of my youthful ambition? He was very different from the type of young man I had been, twenty years before him. And I had had analytic "sons" before. True, I had glimmerings of the way in which his relationship with his

mother and with Ophelia seemed to mirror, or become confused
with, the disintegration of my relationship with my wife. How
deeply wounded I had been to discover Beatrice had been unfaithful to me, how angry! I could never have been unfaithful to her.
She too had changed, like Hamlet, and lost faith in me.

Draw thy breath in pain. . . . I rested my broken arm by the
book on the table in the circular light of the table lamp and
opened with some difficulty a bottle of red wine, meditating on
the possibility that in some way the pain of Hamlet's story was
also the pain of my own story. I needed to approach the one
through the other in order to make any real headway in understanding my unhappiness. What is faith, after all, but the strength
to undergo passionate experience—to approach the unknown, as
Kierkegaard said, in "fear and trembling"? My father, the gentle
Rabbi, had brought me up in the radiance of his own faith—no
refuge for certainties, but exemplifying through spiritual sweet-
ness the tolerance of uncertainties. It was he who told me,

> The three substitutes
> In love for faith
> Are memory, hope
> And sudden death.[1]

My profession, too, has its credo, its articles of faith. Had I not
vowed to receive the fearful strength of the emotion transferred
from the patient's internal objects, with all its gross exaggeration of
the analyst's attributes, giant- or godlike? And in doing so, to also
accept the equal power of the countertransference it evokes—
namely, the parental responsibility, or sense of responsibility, that
enables one to see the child and even the infant in the patient. I
had so vowed; this was the article of faith to which I adhered, the
prerequisite for the operation of the psychoanalytic imagination. I
pondered on some of the well-known modes of breaking faith with
the truth of imagination in my profession—charging exorbitant
fees, exalting common sense, enlisting in the Quality Police—our
modern consumerist version of the Thought Police. I was not, I
thought, guilty of these. There were, indeed, more subtle, more
intimate forms of betrayal—evasions, softenings, glossings over

---

[1] "Faith and Love", a poem by Roland Harris.

the truth. Had there been any such evasions in my handling of Hamlet's analysis, anything that might have contributed to his present regression? I knew I had made mistakes; I had been slow in grasping the significance of his quicksilver changes characteristic of the adolescent mind. But the method allows for this; by the time a new configuration is understood, it has already appeared many times unobserved. The analyst is, after all, always trailing miles behind the patient's unconscious. Hindsight is the very essence of the psychoanalytic method. What can one ever reply to the complaint, "Why didn't you say that before?" One's new idea is already old by the time it can be voiced. There is nothing to be ashamed of in this—it is the only correct, the only effectual position to be in; the method demands it. My allegiance to the method had never faltered. One must have faith in the method and follow its dictates. Was there here any room for doubt?

The claret began to pulse through my veins. I mean *that* wine, Keats's old Wine of Heaven, the redigestion of our most ethereal musings on earth. Hamlet was gone, for ever. In his absence, I had only his story to scrutinize, only my own company in which to digest it. Jesting Pilate could not wait for his answer, but after eight years perhaps the truth was in fact waiting for me, enfolded within Hamlet's story—that journey of recollection that I was about to begin. Already in formulating my quest, I could glimpse the possibility of a different pain at the end of it, the joyful pain of understanding.

> So let me speak to th' yet unknowing world
> How these things came about!
>
> [V. ii. 384–385]

July 1973

Hamlet, the only child of wealthy middle-class parents, was referred to me shortly after his nineteenth birthday for being "impossible" at home: "insufferably rude" and aggressive in his behaviour. His disturbance manifested itself at times in states of extreme withdrawal, during which he would spend hours scribbling in his diary at night, and most of the day asleep, ignoring everybody else in the house. At other times it took the form of wild outbursts of shouting, pushing furniture about, and so on.

One night he had locked his parents out of the house, and they had had to call the police. All this took place when he returned home for the long vacation after his first year reading English at Cambridge University.

* * *

I had had some acquaintance with Hamlet's parents before meeting them to discuss his case. His mother, a gracious and elegant woman of French birth, with liquid dark eyes, was well known for her excellent cuisine and dinner parties, frequented by all the Hampstead intelligentsia. She had a reputation for taking a keen interest in young artists and writers, presiding in effect over a type of literary *salon*. His father was an industrialist, impressive of stature, with gentle green eyes and a wide, sensual, melancholy mouth. He looked, I thought, tired and slightly stooping when I met him this time, while his wife seemed more beautiful than I had remembered. Their worry about Hamlet was exacerbated, they explained, by their total incomprehension. For though they were well aware of adolescent rebellions, negativism, and even breakdowns, there seemed no reason for any of this in Hamlet's case. It was as though he had become an alien being. His hostility seemed particularly directed against his father—to whom, as a young child, he had been very attached.

"Every time he passes Claude on the stairs or wherever (he doesn't eat with us any more, you see)", explained his mother, "he says 'Howdy uncle', or jerks his fingers in some obscene gesture. He really means it, it's most upsetting. After he'd been behaving like this for a while, I told him we'd had enough of his infantile tasteless jokes. Then he gave me such a look, I can't describe it— wild, vicious, almost actual hatred. It was horrible."

While she spoke, Claude winced visibly. Then she added: "And for some time now he's been insulting his father, accusing him of drinking too much—sometimes even in public, either openly or through innuendo. Which is nonsense—Claude drinks socially, like everyone else."

"We do seem to have more social obligations than many people", Claude put in wryly.

"No more than could be helped, with your position and commitments", said his wife to him a little defensively, then, turning to me, she explained that in fact they were trying to cut down on their social engagements, since Claude had had a minor stroke the previous winter. I asked if this had appeared to worry Hamlet.

"Rather the opposite", said his father; "he seems to have taken it as a cue to add to *our* worries." Then he proceeded to explain his own position as a parent: how he was not a domineering father, and Hamlet had never been forced to do anything against his will, nor had unreasonable demands been made of him.

"You must understand, Dr Horacio", he said sorrowfully, "we are not the sort of grossly ambitious parents who would drive their son in some direction that was unsuitable for him. There's no reason for him to turn against us."

"That is very true", confirmed his wife. "All we want is for him to fulfil his own interests in life. We would be perfectly happy if he wanted to become a writer, for example."

"I know what it is to suffer from parental pressures", continued Claude. "It's true that at one time I did hope he'd eventually succeed me in the business. But when it became clear that that was not for him, I never tried to force him into it. I was disappointed, of course. He's a clever boy, we realize that—his teachers have always had great expectations of him. The professor at Cambridge tells us he's one of the most promising students he's ever had."

What about girlfriends? I queried. His mother looked animated: "Now I did suspect it might have something to do with a girlfriend", she said. "Not that Hamlet has ever actually brought a girl home as yet. I thought his diary might give me a clue—he's been writing avidly in it ever since he came home. But these days he keeps it locked. Besides, I thought, this is ridiculous. He's too old to have his secrets prized out that way—what good would it do? No, I thought, if he can't confide in me straightforwardly, then it's better we find him someone else to talk to."

Claude nodded. "Gertrude thinks he needs to let it all out . . . you know . . . in front of somebody other than just the two of us." Then he added, rather furtively, "Do you suppose there's anything you can do about him—I mean, for him?"

I said that I hoped so. Hamlet's symptoms sounded exaggerated but not uncharacteristic of adolescence.

"A type of *normal* madness, you mean?" suggested Claude, "that requires an adjustment of everyone's values, relatively speaking? That's what I used to tell my own father!"

Possibly, I agreed, it could be the degree rather than the kind that exceeded the bounds of the "normal". It was hard to say until I had met him and had seen how he took to working with the psychoanalytic method. Extracting my diary, I said I could offer him three sessions a week, from September on. His parents looked rather astonished. I apologized for only being able to offer three sessions, but pointed out that Hamlet would find it difficult to come down from Cambridge during the term for more than that (he could come, say, on a weekday evening, a Saturday and a Monday morning), and in any case it was always difficult to get adolescents for more than two or three sessions a week.

"Oh, dear—we'd hoped you might be able to discover what was wrong with him before he went back", confessed his mother. Now it was my turn to feel a little stunned. Whatever the nature of his problem, I said, it was bound to involve more than mere diagnosis. Gertrude smiled apologetically and said, "You're quite right, Dr Horacio—we're too impatient. Psychoanalysis isn't an instant cure. That's why it works, isn't it?"

Unfortunately, I had to say, there was never any guarantee of a cure. The very concept of "cure" was no longer considered as valid as it had seemed in the past. But adolescence was always a turbulent and dynamic period, and I was hopeful. Claude asked if they would receive regular progress reports, and I explained that it was not usually appropriate. It was detrimental to the analytic relationship for the child to sense too much conferring behind the scenes; the analyst had to be experienced as an independent figure.

"I see", Claude laughed ruefully; "all I need to do now is pay the monthly bill." He was clearly relieved that somebody else was prepared to take his son's disturbance seriously. Gertrude frowned disapprovingly at him and said she had one more worry: Hamlet was planning to go on a long trekking holiday to India that summer—was he in a fit state of responsibility? This news did rather worry me, and I asked whether he had manifested any other behavioural problems outside his home—at college, for example?

"None that we know of", said his father; "and we know his tutor very well. I'm sure he'd have told us if he'd noticed anything. All he ever says is how delighted he is with Hamlet's progress, in fact with everything about Hamlet." With mournful irony, he added, "Hamlet is the apple of his eye."

In that case, I replied (somewhat helplessly), it would probably be reasonable for him to go; I imagined it would be impossible to stop him anyway—was he going alone?

"No", said Gertrude, "he's going with a friend, someone we've known for ages—the son of his tutor, Professor Polack, in fact. He's a bit older than Hamlet, and he's been before. I wouldn't necessarily call him more responsible, though, in the normal way of things."

"They'll be all right", said Claude decisively. "It will do him good."

After the Danes had left, I meditated on the strong appeal of their personal qualities—their modesty and openness. This was the first private conversation I had had with either of them, though I too had been to their parties and been impressed by the glittering ambience of highly tasteful cultured wealth and manners. Undoubtedly I was younger than many of the psychoanalysts with whom they had contact; but instinctively, I felt, they had chosen someone eager to respond to the challenge of their troublesome son. It was an interesting fact, I reflected (not for the first time), that even children of the most sensitive and devoted parents, brought up in conditions of privilege, were still not immune to psychological disturbance.

I had one preliminary interview with Hamlet himself before the summer holiday. He was one of those teenagers who are clearly unhappy on their feet: he arrived at my house in Flask Walk on a bike, which he leant unlocked against the railings just outside the semi-basement window of my consulting-room. He loped down the steps and rang. Being just on time for his appointment, I admitted him directly, and he sat down on the chair in the corner of the room, whence he could scan, simultaneously, the bike, the couch and myself. I was struck by his resemblance to his mother—an angular and lanky version of her poised and graceful figure, with identical dark eyes, though his were half hidden by long and greasy locks of hair. For a couple of minutes he darted an occasional hawk-like glance at me from behind his hair.

"I expect you'll say you can't psychoanalyse me unless I lie on the couch", he commenced. "Well, I'm afraid I'm not going to, because to my mind nothing could be more ridiculous."

I reassured him that this was simply an introductory meeting, and there was no hurry to use the couch until he felt ready to do so. The function of the couch was to help him collect his thoughts and associations, free from the distraction of looking at me, the analyst. I gave my usual explanation of my way of working with the psychoanalytic method: the discipline of the routine, the setting, the fifty-minute sessions, and so on; the importance of trying to be frank in relating whatever came into his mind during the session, however absurd it might seem, rather than storing up things to tell me outside the sessions; above all, the importance of trying to remember his dreams. At this last, a wave of panic clouded his eyes beneath the hair, and he assured me he didn't dream and certainly couldn't remember his dreams. "And as for telling you all the things that might cross my mind while I'm sitting here, I can't imagine anything more boring. It'd be like trying to write an essay without giving it a moment's thought—just scribbling one word after another."

In practice, I said, he would find that only things relevant to the analytic situation (that is, the emotional situation) would come to his mind. That was the beauty of the method. All I required was for him to relate them honestly to me.

He parted a strand of hair over one eye and peered intensely at me: "You really are weird", he said. "What a peculiar idea—to call a method beautiful—even if it is a method, and I don't see that it is a method at all. Not a scientific method."

I commented that, inevitably, this was something he would come to understand only with experience. He seemed a little stung by this minor rebuke and said condescendingly:

"You'll find I know a lot more about this business than my uncle does. He's never given it a thought till he got it into his head to send me here. He's desperate to get rid of me, you see. As a matter of fact", he added provocatively, "I *put* it into his head. I'm interested in expanding my mind."

He paused, eyeing me for effect. Why his "uncle"? I asked.

"Uncle Claude, of course", he said in a matter-of-fact tone, but with a defiant, piercing stare. "You've met him, haven't you?"

"Ah", I said, and then asked Hamlet what he had found out about psychoanalysis.

"Well", he began to chatter, "I've read quite a bit to start with—introductions to the various schools and things—I got a reading list from my Director of Studies, he's really into all that. That's just background, of course. Then I've got a couple of friends who've actually been psychoanalysed. Rosenfeld's still having his complexes sorted out—he had a terrible childhood, his parents just dumped him at school. He used to come into the prefects' common-room at lunchtime, after his session, and tell us what else they'd discovered about what his parents had done to his primary processes before his memory became conscious. He was having a Freudian analysis, but Gildstein—my other friend—had a Kleinian one, so I got the chance to compare the two. Gildstein's mother actually is a psychoanalyst, so he had it prophylactically when he was quite young, to stop him getting anything later. The Kleinians believe in prevention rather than cure, don't they— aren't you a Kleinian?"

Under cover of his naivety (and I couldn't quite make out whether this was genuine or assumed), he was giving the impression of a cat waiting to pounce. I realized I would have to be on my guard with this Elephant's Child. I pointed out that his friends' stories still came into the category of hearsay (or "background", as he called it), and he should be prepared to find his own experience rather different. But, since he had clearly made some inquiries about *my* background, I asked him what other information he had discovered about me?

"You're a great writer of scientific papers, aren't you", he replied immediately. (Oh, dear, I thought.) When I asked if he had read any, he replied "Well, sort of. Can't say I was impressed by your style—too much jargon. And some of your ideas are a bit old-fashioned. But yeah—it was OK" (he said, drumming his fingers on his knee). "But I'm surprised the people you're writing about let you get away with it—exposing all their secrets in public like that."

I saw he was convinced that I would want to write a "scientific paper" about him, and also nervous about my doing so. I explained that such papers were written for other clinical practitioners and had a very limited circulation and intelligibility, and that the identity of patients was protected by altering names and other features.

"Names! What's in a *name*?" he exclaimed contemptuously, as if I were either very casual or very credulous. "You wouldn't be able to write anything about me, with my parentage, without everybody knowing exactly who you were talking about. 'Oh yes now, the Dane boy', they'll be gossiping behind their whisky glasses, 'he's been seeing Dr Horacio lately; now you know what his problem turns out to be . . .' blah blah blah."

I caught an early glimpse here of the grandiosity, in its attention-seeking context, which was to prove a central problem in the analysis; and already it worried me. To defuse it, I explained to Hamlet that there was also a more subtle form of protection, founded on the nature of the psychoanalytic relationship and the "countertransference" of the analyst's reception of the patient's feelings, which meant that it was understood the analyst was always writing subjectively—and, in essence, about himself. He grinned as he took this in.

"Oh, very good", he said. "I like it—real slippery, man. So nobody gets to find out the real secret after all."

It was, rather, I said, that the concept of their being "a secret" was a mistaken one. It was better to think of the mind as "having mystery" than as "hiding secrets".

"Oh, yeah?" he taunted suspiciously. "You're not religious or anything, are you?"

The psychoanalytic method, I told him, was designed to focus on mental events—thoughts, feelings, the organization and interaction of internal figures or objects. These were difficult to observe and understand, which was why we relied so much on dreams to "tell the truth" about an internal situation.

"I don't see how psychoanalysis can cure if it can't even find out what's wrong", he said, "whether you call it a secret or a mystery."

I agreed that our goal was better defined as observing, clarifying, understanding, than "curing". He meditated on this for a moment and then concluded that that, of course, was exactly why he had come—not to be cured (it was not as though there were anything wrong with him) but to "investigate his inner mystery".

On his way out he noticed that I held out my hand, and he gave it a hurried and embarrassed shake. This initial meeting made an enduring impression on me. I was touched by his eagerness to "investigate" himself and by his willingness to view me almost immediately as someone to whom he could attach a child-like dependence. He had been ready, almost before seeing me, to adopt me as the real friend whom he evidently felt he lacked. It was clear that he had motivated his parents to seek out an analyst for him. But I was worried, also, by a certain fixedness in his attitude: he had a preformed idea of my function as an analyst and how I would serve him; and, above all, it seemed clear that the confusion about his "uncle–father" had the fixed structure of a delusion, with its attendant danger of incipient schizophrenia.

For his first analytic session, some two months later, Hamlet arrived on his bike as before and entered the consulting-room with a busy, eager air, wearing a long blue Indian shirt, patched jeans, and sandals. He had a newly grown beard. He glanced around and nodded at me, as though my presence in the room were a fortuitous event—one more accident befalling him on his travels. Then, rather to my surprise, he flung himself down on the couch and began to talk animatedly, moving his arms, about the people and events that had filled his summer holidays. He had gone to India with a friend named Nando ("short for Ferdinand—his father's Italian"), and the account of their travels (which I realized I was not the first to listen to) was clearly embellished and glamorized with each successive telling, though it included spending a week prostrate with severe diarrhoea and, on the way home, two nights in a Turkish jail under suspicion of drug trafficking. This last was recounted as if it were the highlight of a royal tour from which his return was eagerly awaited.

"Rosenfeld and Gildstein are back too", he announced meaningfully, turning his head from the couch as though to clinch his demonstration that his entire court now surrounded him. (Needless to say, I had only the haziest recollection of who Rosenfeld and Gildstein might be.)

The air of prickly awkwardness that had characterized Hamlet on our original meeting had vanished. But there was no sign, either, of the few moments of emotional contact. I gathered I was supposed to be impressed by his new man-of-the-world bearing; and as I was pondering on this, he broke off his narration and accused me of not listening:

"I suppose you're really only interested in my sex life", he said provocatively.

I replied that I would like to hear more about his friend Nando—had he known him long?

"For ever", he yawned. "He was rugby captain at school—the year above me. Yeah, he's a great one for boasting about his sexual exploits—you guessed. Nando's all right, though. It was OK going away with him, you knew he wouldn't leave you in the lurch." (This was the first indication that there could have been any "lurches".) "He's into transcendental meditation and all that. He shares a house with some friends now, in Islington. He's left home. His dad's my supervisor at Cambridge—though you'd never believe Nando was sired by an intellectual wizard."

The intellectual wizard, Professor Polack, was to figure prominently in the analysis, as would all the members of the Polack family. His schoolboy homosexual relationship with Nando was soon to transfer to an intense involvement with his sister Ophelia. I learned that Hamlet had in fact known the family since childhood, and until recently had been at school with Nando, who had stayed on as a boarder when his father and sister moved to Cambridge. From his first year as a student Hamlet had been filled with an intense admiration for the Professor, and, as far as I could gather, this seemed to be more or less reciprocated. Meanwhile I was told the "amazing" history of Polack's arrival in England. An Italian Jew whose father had been "something high up in politics" before the war, his original name was Polaco. When the war came, all his family were killed in concentration camps, and he only survived because an English girl helped him to escape—via ox-carts, guards'-vans, and the bilge of a fishing boat—until she got him to England and married him. She died when the children were very young, and the Professor brought them up on his own—according to Hamlet, heroically concentrating on their education:

"It cost him a fortune to keep Nando at school, you know. As for Ophelia, he had her made into a fabulous musician—she can play anything from the cello to a host of weird medieval instruments. Come to think of it", he added, "they've both had far more attention showered on them than my parents ever paid me."

Here was a surprising departure, I thought—hadn't he been given opportunities by his parents that were at least the equivalent of the Polack children's?

"Conventionally speaking, maybe", he acquiesced rather pompously. "But not in real terms. I was just supposed to fit the bill—come top in exams, bow and scrape to the guests at home, make polite conversation—do my stuff, however skewiff and screwed up I felt inside. The performing dog." Then he explained, confidentially, "I expect the early death of his wife helped. That meant he could bring Nando and Ophelia up the way he wanted—no interference."

It was interesting, I commented ironically, that a feature of Hamlet's grievance was that he had two parents instead of one— implying that mothers were not really necessary, just background. He spoke as though his two parents, being conjoined in some confusing way, had somehow prevented his being "thought about" such that he could develop upwards in a clean straight line, as Ophelia had grown straight up into a musician. By contrast he, Hamlet, felt he was growing all "skewiff".

At this he turned on me with a sudden vehemence and said, "OK, so I've been lumbered with a whole load of inherited problems—my uncle, for a start! Anyone can see what a debauched, drunken, degenerate old lecher he is—yet my mother thinks the sun shines out of his arse. But I could tolerate that if it wasn't for the hypocrisy and vanity of them all! The trouble with adults is, they can't understand the difference between training and education. They want their children to 'perform well' . . . yes, like dogs . . . and for whose sake? Certainly not the child's. Look at me—I haven't been 'brought up', I've been bred—like a horse on a prize stud farm—groomed in everything from table manners to socialist politics. And it's all for their own vanity and self-satisfaction . . . at best . . . and at worst it's so they can show off to the neighbours at the next dinner party!"

I was taken aback and rather stung by this outburst. Clearly Hamlet was accusing me of being one of the adult "trainers" who merely wished to bring him into line for their egotistical satisfaction. I remembered the time when I had made a similar distinction about training and education to my own father, although—I be-lieve—in a less hurtful manner (I never really quarrelled with him). I told Hamlet he was complaining about institutional val-ues—the "stud farm"—as a way of ignoring the more complex problems associated with intimate relationships, such as with his parents. In rejecting these as institutional, so beneath his notice, he was avoiding their real difficulties.

"It's they who think we're beneath *their* notice", retorted Ham-let. "The standard adult line is that children can be seen and heard, but only saying the right things. And they're quite oblivi-ous to the fact that the children might be seeing and hearing *them*. No—*they're* the ones who are always playing at secrets, because they can't tell the difference between a secret and a mystery!"

He was an interesting boy, I thought, after this little alterca-tion. There was more perspicacity in his criticism of the adult world than in the standard adolescent defiance, and at the same time more delusion. His mother was seen to be tainted by her adhesiveness to his contemptible "uncle"–father, who had himself been split off from his "real" father. Presumably he had ensconced himself in the Professor's affections as an alternative to this. I began to form a picture of the seriously entrenched nature of Hamlet's grandiosity—his overpowering need to show off and be admired, to be indeed the prize horse in the stud. Thus, at one session, he was full of how he had just been to dinner at Polack's house, along with some other students, and been the life and soul of the party owing to his satirical impersonations of public figures, which had delighted the Professor. This was recounted in the midst of other social triumphs: the engineering of crushing blows against the establishment, such as forcing the college authorities to install a condom machine in the toilet, or to provide a photocopy-ing machine for the JCR, on the grounds of equality of dissemina-tion of information.

The session after this, he brought me an interesting little dream, which illuminated the tongue-in-cheek nature of his ideal-ized view of the Polack family relationships. The dream began with *a birds'-eye view of a glittering blue ocean, in the midst of which was a small speck. Gradually this came into nearer focus (as in a film) and showed itself to be a tiny picture-postcard island, with a ring of yellow sand and coconut palms. In the middle of the ring stood Professor*

Polack, dressed like a children's magician in a huge purple cloak span-
gled with stars and moons, his arms upraised, with a wand in one hand
and his bald head with its pointed beard looking upwards to the sky.
"I realized he was saying something, as if he was casting a spell. He
seemed to be saying, 'Grow, my children; grow, and prosper!' Then I
could see that there was a big white cloud above his head, soft and puffy
against the blue sky, like those rococo ceilings. And Nando and Ophelia
were sitting cross-legged in the centre of the cloud, dressed in gold and
white kaftans, putting chocolates in each other's mouths."

Hamlet seemed amused by this dream, saying it was like a
mixture of chocolate and insurance adverts. "It's a classic wish-
fulfilment dream", he pronounced ". . . wish-fulfilment for adults,
that is. They produce this scenario exactly like an advert and
put the children in the middle to act out their fantasies for them.
Now children—grow up nicely, and be a credit to your doting
parents. What good children, taking their exams and eating their
chocolates! 'Prosper'—that's a pun on status-making, of course.
Aristocratic pretensions, all of them."

Yes, I agreed, this dream showed us his underlying mockery
of the Professor's methods of upbringing, in which the entire
adult world was implicated. In Hamlet's view, the Professor with
his wand thinks he is "raising" the children, handing down wis-
dom—ignorant that secretly (including through sexual games) the
children are really raising themselves.

But as well as Hamlet's mockery of the Professor's self-ideali-
zation and the complicity of brother and sister in it, the dream
also suggested his essential loneliness as an only child who had
no one in the family with whom to share his childishness—only
adults.

Hamlet then told me of a strange vision, or memory-flash, he
had had the other day when sitting with Nando and his friends
doing transcendental meditation "for a laugh". An image of
Ophelia from some years before had come vividly to his mind. In
this, she was sitting perched on her brother's shoulders during a
political demonstration; it was one of the few occasions he had
seen her in London since she had moved to Cambridge.

"She was wearing a green duffle-coat, with her long fair hair
falling right down over his face. Her mouth was very pink; it kept
opening and shutting, and the air was grey and frosty. Her breath

was rising up in clouds. She was chanting rhythmically, 'pigs go home'. She looked really angry, kind of transported."

I asked Hamlet whether the Polack brother and sister were particularly good-looking, to which he assented rather casually (sounding surprised), adding that Nando had sometimes been nicknamed "Adonis" at school. "But she's more talented than he is", he corrected me, lest I should imagine he was swayed by such superficial characteristics as physical beauty.

The image, I suggested, implied that Nando had the body and Ophelia the brains of their brother–sister combination.

"Nando's not stupid", said Hamlet, "he's just not academic."

Nevertheless I suspected that Hamlet's hero-worship of the rugger-captain Adonis–Nando had a rather tentative quality, as did his idealization of his "magician" father. I also noted there was something a little unsavoury about the sister, with her "pigs go home"—who were the pigs?

"I dunno", said Hamlet nonchalantly, "police, I suppose . . . can't remember."

This was in a sense the underside to the chocolate picture—showing how the children had the upper hand, were the driving force of the adult world. Again, there seemed to be something of Hamlet's own infancy in it. Thinking of Hamlet's solitary childhood, I asked him whether there might be any connection with riding on his father's shoulders when he was very young. He agreed with surprise that he could remember doing that. And I described to him the glimpse I now had of the boy–Hamlet, elevated by his father's stature yet believing that he had elevated himself and was in fact the only real king, directing and controlling his father's movements.

We parted after this session with a mutual wary respect. I had a much clearer idea of the seriousness of his problem—his grandiosity, with its infantile roots in his relationship with his father, and the delusional form it had now taken with the despised "uncle–father" who was no longer responsive to his direction and to the mutual idealization he demanded. At the same time I was impressed, and surprised, by his cooperativeness and eagerness—different from the usual aggression and antagonism of the adolescent. I was stirred by both his incisiveness and his dependence. For underneath his contempt for the follies of the adult world, I could sense strongly the lonely child's nostalgia for being Daddy's boy. Perhaps this spoke to me more readily as I had no son and felt this a gap in my life. Already I could foresee a pattern of transference relationships forming in which I knew I should have to tread carefully. In the intensity of Hamlet's desire to explore his mystery and to be admired, something he had attached to Polack—and previously to his father—was already beginning to transfer itself to me.

The Ghost

GHOST:　If thou has nature in thee, bear it not,
　　　　Let not the royal bed of Denmark be
　　　　A couch for luxury and damned incest.
　　　　But howsomever thou pursuest this act,
　　　　Taint not thy mind, nor let thy soul contrive
　　　　Against thy mother aught.

[I. v. 82–86]

The week after this, Hamlet brought me a fascinating and crucial dream, whose mirroring of deep emotional conflicts would prove central to the analysis for a long time. The "Ghost Dream" became a major point of reference for us.

In this dream, *Hamlet saw his father in his fighter-pilot's uniform from the war, seated inside his Spitfire wearing flying suit and goggles. He seemed larger than life, surrounded by a shimmering golden aura, and the plane's wings seemed to be quivering in a violent wind. Their shadow enveloped Hamlet as he stood outside the plane and shivered. Hamlet felt tiny by contrast with his father in the plane, and intimidated.*

Above all, he felt bewildered and wanted desperately to know what was happening, and he cried out:

> *"Let me not burst in ignorance! Why do you*
> *Shake my nature with such awesome thoughts*
> *Beyond the utmost reaching of my soul?*
> *Say why! What should I think? What must I do?"*

At this point his father raised his goggles to reveal his face, and moved his lips in reply, though his voice itself was inaudible and its sound seemed to be transferred through the beating of the plane's wings. In this way, Hamlet heard his father's complaint about his own unhappiness and its history:

> *"O Hamlet! the secrets of my prison-house*
> *Are the fruits of lust, your mother's lust,*
> *That seeming-virtuous angel whose sweet milk*
> *Turned all to sourness and to sadness—a drink*
> *Most serpentine—the day she treacherously*
> *Abandoned me by weaning as I lay*
> *On Lethe's wharf, and rooted at my ease.*
> *Placidly rocking and unsuspecting, I was*
> *Ignorant that her desires had turned*
> *Elsewhere."*

Hamlet noticed that his father was turning to start the plane for takeoff. So again he asked urgently what he should "do", and his father said in the same ghostly tones, transmitted through vibrations in the wind,

> *"Remember me, my son! and seek revenge.*
> *But however you choose to set about it, never*
> *Taint your mind, nor harm your mother at all."*

Then the noise of the engine drowned all other sounds as the plane began to move down the runway. But first it circled Hamlet three times, and he noticed painted on the plane's nose the seductive image of a girl in bathing costume, and the name in twirly lettering, "Gertrude".

I was thrilled with the imaginative richness of this dream, with its direct—if ambiguous—focusing on Hamlet's troubled relationship with his father, and having his mother as a key gravitational force in the background, both attracting and repelling. The dream certainly had a glamorous quality, which Hamlet associated with his father's decorations for bravery that hung in the lobby of their home, in a corner devoted to more formal mementoes of family history, including photographs of his parents' wedding and of his father standing by his plane in wartime. In this sense the dream showed his father-as-hero, protecting his mother or mother country from invasion in the war. At the same time it showed him his aggressiveness towards women—relating this to the infant at weaning, feeling abandoned by this wife/mother at the same time as becoming conscious of his dependence on her.

This father, whose ambiguity stemmed from his ambiguous internal picture of womanhood, seemed to transfer his own quandary to Hamlet in the dream. Hamlet himself was excluded from the dizzy sexual heights (and dangers) attained by the plane (with his mother's name); his father was taking off without him. But, I wondered, mulling over his father's final words, in what precise sense was the model of sexuality he presented one of "revenge"?

"It's revenge on my mother for taking up with Uncle Claude, of course", pronounced Hamlet, who had been listening to my ruminations with an air of bemused impatience. "There's something shameful, at her age, about the way she fusses and fawns all over him—even more since he's been ill. It's degraded, when you consider what my father was like—but she's only got herself to blame!"

I asked him to explain to me the difference between his "father" and "Uncle Claude". He responded eagerly, as though at last he'd been given the opportunity to set this straight:

"Things were quite different before Uncle Claude took over. Everybody admired my father—he was generous, idealistic, strong. There was nothing sneaky or underhand about him, everything was open and aboveboard. He was the kind of man who, if he had lived, would really have made a difference to society—because he meant what he said, and he would have carried it out. Not like Claude . . ." (and here he began to list scornfully the evidence, in his eyes, of his father's physical and mental decay—his illness, drinking too heavily, problems of finance and industrial relations at the chemical factory which he owned and managed and had built up from nothing.) "And now he is being investigated by the Inland Revenue. So much for being a respectable capitalist with socialist principles! I suppose he thought he could get away for ever with having it both ways. It just shows—if he's not screwing a woman he's screwing the workers. Yuck. Degeneration in mind and body."

I saw that in Hamlet's mind his father literally seemed to have become someone else—though still a close relative, the "brother" of his former self. The wartime captain of nobility and heroism, and genuine socialist beliefs, had been exchanged for the usurping industrial chief. I asked him at what point this transformation seemed to have taken place, and he said he couldn't remember precisely because he must have been quite young, but he remembered vividly when the truth of what had happened first began to dawn upon him, when he was thirteen or fourteen. At that time he began to think for himself—his eyes were opened, and he regretted having gone along with his mother in pretending that there was nothing wrong, because then it became crystal clear to him what a mess this weak hypocritical ploy had made of their family relationships.

"That's what's so pathetic about the older generation", said Hamlet in a bitterly scathing tone; "adults think they're so clever at hiding secrets from children, even when it's blatantly obvious to everyone what's going on!"

I said it was Hamlet's conviction that his mother, well-intentioned but foolish, had kept his father's death when he was a young child a secret from him, hoping that he wouldn't remember and that Claude would be a completely satisfactory stepfather for him. Without making any direct reply to this interpretation, he continued even more vigorously, as though more evidence was required to convince me of his mother's folly:

"The end result is, it's *me* who has to tell *her* what she's doing wrong—because it's only herself she manages to blind. You see, Dr Horacio, my mother thought she could cover it all over by holding court in her drawing-room, surrounded by sycophants and flatterers—the best class of people, of course, with impeccable views on politics and culture—all enviously grateful for being allowed to participate in such scintillating conversation and to swill booze with Claude from the cellar that never runs dry. Life with the Danes—pillars of society and civilization on the surface, and a rotting dungheap of social climbers underneath!"

Returning to the dream, whose rich "cellar" of imagery I felt we had only begun to tap, I showed him how the image of his father-as-hero now demanded adjustment in the light of his own adolescent turbulence, including his jaundiced view of the adult world now his "eyes were opened".

"All that aeroplane stuff, of course", said Hamlet dismissively, "belongs to when I was a little boy and was mad about planes and wanted to be a pilot myself. That makes this dream outdated in a way. None of that turns me on any more, obviously. A Ghost–pilot from the past."

The dream, however, I pointed out, was about "now", not about "then". The hero–father who had returned like a ghost from the past history of his boyhood ideals now seemed to be introducing him to the anxieties of adulthood. These were looming over him like the wings of his father's aeroplane. In particular, he was being introduced to his own ambivalence towards women, by a father whose role seemed to be that of both protector and conqueror. This upsurgence within himself was what was now troubling him.

"It seems to me that *they're* the ones who are in trouble", said Hamlet with a casual disdain, ignoring my interpretation of his personal conflict. "They should have a health warning written all over them—'Avoid my example—I'm obsolete.' They just can't adjust to the way things are now. In the war it was all right and wrong, good and bad. United goals and jolly camaraderie—with God on their side. That was easy. Now they've lost their sense of direction and it's all wheeling and dealing, shuffling and committee meetings. Bribery and corruption. Drink and debauchery."

Hamlet's persistent, and perspicacious, variation on the usual adolescent theme of how the children had long discovered everything the adults had tried to hide from them, was that the adults themselves were really children without knowing it. Nevertheless I wanted to remind him of his own personal helplessness, which had been clearly expressed in the dream as "bursting in ignorance".

"Yeah, maybe", he drawled, more aggressively, "but the fact is it's us lot—the new generation—who are going to be lumbered with sorting *them* out."

The dream, I stressed, showed that the first place he needed to look to begin to "sort things out" was inside himself, at his own internal condition. Instead of attributing blame to his internal father-and-mother, he needed to locate the positive qualities they could offer to help him work through his own conflicts.

"Internal father and mother! They look a pretty insalubrious pair to me", he mocked. "Status and Self-gratification—that's their scene in a nutshell."

Status and self-gratification, I agreed, could certainly be defined as unhelpful qualities, which could take "revenge" on him and distort his mental growth. Our job in the analysis was to disentangle these from the genuinely parental qualities to be found in his internal objects.

"Oh yeah—disentangle! I like it!" he sneered. "The fact is, when you get right down to it—no one wants a feller with a social disease."

I half-recognized this reference, and he expounded for me: "You know—Officer Krupke—it's what they say to him in *West Side Story*:

"Our mothers all are junkies,
Our fathers all are drunks—
Goodness gracious!
Naturally we're punks."

He concluded, addressing me slyly as he left, "OK, Officer Krupke?"

I pondered, after he had gone, on his quick switches of attitude to me and these other parental figures. At one moment he would cooperate with me, as much in the sense of conspiring as of being helped (with a definite element of showing-off); the next moment, I was relegated to being some constricting "authority" figure. My technique with him was not made easier by his innate deftness at twisting our conversation into the form of a debate—a form with which he obviously felt familiar and in control, and where winning his point took precedence over confronting the truth about himself. He had a natural talent for avoiding the intimate emotionality with which my interpretations tried to bring him in touch. And yet, it was all there in his dream! Once again, I admired its richness. The Ghost Dream was to be the first in a series of imaginative dreams that astounded me by their emotional depth and awareness, each time inspiring me with new hope even when in the depths of despondency.

It was, however, a strange phenomenon—that despite his perspicacity, even brilliance, Hamlet did not seem to have grasped the concept of learning from an individual, or of being taught by them. His immediate attachment to me—from our first meeting— had an automatic quality, not a reciprocal quality founded on real appreciation and the growth of trust in me. This made me think of the Professor, who, I suspected, now filled the gap left by Hamlet's early idealization of his father. And, in turn, I was reminded of certain troubling factors in my own life: anxiety about the prospect of my daughters' adolescence; the vague sense that my wife and I had drifted apart; above all, regret that I had no son. My countertransference involvement with Hamlet made me acutely conscious of all these factors, especially the last. Had I, perhaps, idealized Hamlet's parents, leaping to conclusions about their excellence, as a way of escaping my own anxieties and problems in this difficult and unsatisfactory sphere? Was there more truth in his criticism of them than I had cared to investigate? I worried, as I did recurrently with other patients, whether I tended to get too involved with my analytic work, investing too much personal emotion in it at the expense of my home life.

Meanwhile, over the next few days, my reflections returned to Hamlet's relationship with his new substitute-father, the Professor, and I wondered how it would progress. I was curious to observe its evolution. But before I heard more about this, Hamlet's sudden intimacy with the Professor's daughter burst in on the analysis, taking me by surprise with its intensity and rapidity.

One evening, Hamlet came in curiously garbed, with a profusion of chains and bangles worn over his leather jacket with its collar up, and dark glasses propped above his forehead (he had by now shaved his beard). I was struck immediately by a resemblance to the Ghost–pilot of his dream and remarked that his armoury gave him an inaccessible appearance. He countered sharply:

"It isn't me that's inaccessible. It's that frigid tart. She is avoiding me—not entirely (that would at least be honest), but she won't come out with me alone. As it is, I see her almost every day, but always surrounded by a bodyguard of friends, or her father. Or else she's 'got to work'."

Who is this? I interrupted—Polack's daughter?

"Yes, Ophelia!" he snapped irritably. "Last night I dreamed *I flew into her window—a sort of Batman act, storming the citadel—and had her:*

> *Heaving a sigh so piteous and profound*
> *It seemed to shatter all my bulk*
> *And end my being.*

And after the dream, of course, I realized that that was just how she wanted it—that's what would fulfil her feminine fantasies! That's the way they all like to see themselves—swept up like the princess in the tower, all virginal and starry-eyed. And that, of course", he added with a savage cynicism, "is their prescription for how it's got to seem to be, whatever the dirty realities might be underneath it all!"

Hamlet then explained, in response to my query, that Ophelia did not live at home with her father, though she was often there at weekends, but had a room at her women's college—an "institution like a nunnery"—and her window was on the second floor, as in the dream. However, he had no intention of shinning up a drainpipe like Romeo: "The hypocrisy of the whole affair! That's what's so disgusting. I don't mean only her, but everybody. No men are allowed in there after 11 at night, which simply means there's a man stowed in every cupboard. And I'm only interested in equal sex, not some archaic fantasy of wooing and conquering. What the hell's the point of pretending to worship virginity these days? This isn't the Edwardian era. Yet we still haven't caught up with Shaw's diagnosis—we haven't learned to separate all the paraphernalia of marriage contracts etc. (which are simply designed to perpetuate social hierarchies) from the itch in the flesh which should be honestly viewed for what it is. It's time the cobwebs were swept away and some clear thinking was introduced."

It was the first time I had seen Hamlet in the full flow of a ranting rage, though it was not to be the last. It was a curious phenomenon—unleashed, as I took it, by the "Ghost" within him.

"It's all pretence anyway!" he added, with renewed vehemence. "When you get right down to it—behind all the simpering
and fluttering of eyelashes. Whatever age they are, it's the same
story. Look at my mother, with her wretched parties and her host-
ess act—pretending it's her social duty to flirt and gratify all the
little whims of her goggling guests. She'd like to make out it's all
part of the patronage system, all 'doing good'. The reality is, all
women are secret whores. You—I suppose—would call it female
masochism. It's innate. It's no different with Ophelia and all her
fake-modest smiling and nodding. Does she think I'm some ignorant fool, who doesn't know anything about her past or—for that
matter—her present goings-on? Or doesn't she care, so long as the
façade of worshipful courtship is paced out in the approved manner, like some strutting peacock?"

I was impressed by the impact Ophelia seemed to have made
on him, which I had certainly not expected from his earlier detached, quizzical descriptions of a rather withdrawn figure who
had seemed a mere appendage of her brother. I found myself
suddenly curious to know what she was really like. Again I
showed Hamlet his identification with the aggressive aspect of the
Ghost–pilot—as it appeared in his "Batman" Dream, his contemptuous speech about women as "secret whores", and indeed his
own clothing. This was the domineering and status-conscious side
of the fighter-pilot rather than the protective side. The implication
seemed to be that his father, with his old-fashioned methods of
"wooing and conquering", would have no difficulty in flying
through "paraphernalia" and "cobwebs"—in fact, would have
known how to make use of them as part of his own equipment for
satisfying this "itch in the flesh".

"That's Claude's obsession, more like", observed Hamlet sarcastically. "But Claude's methods are more slimy, less energetic.
And my mother panders to him, all the more to compensate for
her flirting with the other riffraff. She's a fool."

The Batman Dream should be taken as a warning, I said. It
showed us the significance of acting-out, dressing up to imitate
the Ghost–pilot–daddy, indeed, getting inside this aggressive
aeroplane–daddy and his penis in the sense of a weapon. We
could understand better now what had at first been puzzling in
the Ghost's mention of "revenge". The concept of revenge, I re-

minded him, had come up in response to Hamlet's reiterated question about what he should "do". Revenge was the answer to the desire for action—demonstrated clearly in the Batman Dream.

"Surely", objected Hamlet, "the point is, what *kind* of action? You can't say all action is bad, all action is vengeful. You might as well say all sex is bad, so all we are allowed to do is think about it."

The distinction presented by the dreams, I explained, was a very fundamental one between "action" and "communication". Action was really acting-out—acting on somebody or their feelings, manipulating them. In the Batman Dream, for example, there was clearly no intention to communicate anything to Ophelia, but simply to conquer by action.

"That's because I knew *she'd* want it that way", he protested. "Like all women, she's a devout romancer. It goes with deviousness. I told you, I don't go for that primitive bullshit myself, it's ludicrous. You don't believe the height of my ambition is to play Batman in the movies, do you?" he sneered.

As a dream-image, I said, it was no more ludicrous than that of the Ghost–pilot. It conveyed a meaning, which need not be literally translated into shinning up a drainpipe—there were other forms of "action" on Ophelia that he might find himself taking. Or possibly on his mother, as the Ghost had suggested; for we seemed to be dealing generally with the question of his attitude to women. The Ghost's implication was that, motivated by revenge against women, he might "taint" his own mind. This was the sort of action we needed to guard against.

"Honestly, Dr Horacio, you have such an overdramatic view of my character", said he condescendingly. "You'd think I went around with a pocketful of hand-grenades. Consider—I am a peace-loving intellectual. I only fight when justifiably aroused— even at school that was my reputation. Nobody can call me a coward—but I'm not an aggressor either. And certainly not against women! *But*", he added on a harsh and ugly note, "neither am I prepared to be played on by Ophelia's goody-goody masochism. I'm not going to be teased into acting the sadist just to satisfy her feminine fancies! She can bloody well take me as I am or not at all."

Uneasy at his unwillingness to be put in touch with the violence of his own feelings, I stressed again the importance of continuously examining his own motives in terms of action versus communication. And this time, instead of replying instantly, he reached into his jacket pocket and extracted—not a hand-grenade, but a folded piece of paper.

"I can see", he announced, "that nothing less than the oracular proof will satisfy you. Shall I read you the poem I sent Ophelia? Then you'll see that I do nothing without communication."

He rather caught me by surprise, and I began to demur, but he interrupted: "Don't worry, it's not just a private love-letter—it's a poem, so it's universal, you can make what you like of it. In fact, it's going into *Varsity* next week." And hastily he began to recite:

> "O fuck, fuck, fuck,
> you play on me, and seem to know my
> stops.
> But if only my finger and tongue could
> govern your ventages,
> you'd see what excellent music would sound
> from the top to the bottom
> from this little organ
> at the heart of my
> mystery."

My heart was sinking as he read. I imagined he must be having a pretty offputting effect on Ophelia, and I was anxious to enable him to find some way of containing himself. The poem itself, I told him, was a good illustration of what we had been talking about— it was action disguised as communication. This was his translation into real life of the action of the Batman Dream: the "fuck, fuck" aspect of himself, which believed that all it had to do was "govern the ventages".

"How can you say that", he complained, sounding somewhat crushed, "when it's a straightforward plea for an equal relationship?"

In an equal relationship, I said, neither person should be merely a pipe to be played on; it would be necessary to imagine the other person, also, as having "mystery". At the beginning of the session he had leapt to conclusions about "hypocrisy" instead of admitting that he didn't understand Ophelia's intentions towards him. But instead of trying to gauge her state of mind, he had allowed himself to become inflamed and to "act the Ghost" by means of this letter.

"You just don't like the sexual explicitness in the poetic ambiguity", he declared, recovering his poise. "It's too modern for your taste. You wouldn't mind if it was a dream, but you think a poem should be censored."

I realized then that it was no use his bringing his poems here for interpretation as if they were dreams; in fact, it was probably counterproductive. I explained that his poetry was liable to be censored or arranged by himself, whereas a dream could speak directly to us about the processes of his inner world. For our purposes, a dream was explicit and a poem was not.

"Well, if you don't approve of 'arranging' material", he countered accusingly, "perhaps you should consider more closely what it is that you're doing with my dreams when you put them in one of your scientific papers! Aren't you just arranging them to suit yourself? I suppose you want to be the only person credited with talent."

The dream, I explained, was always his dream, as he had reported it, in no way tampered with; my interpretation of it and of the whole analytic situation could perhaps be called my dream of his dream. This was the case here and now, just as much as in scientific papers, should I ever include his material in those.

"Your dream", he repeated, with a guarded, surly spark of interest", "that's more like it, yeah!"

Nevertheless, he spent the last minutes of the session in a huff, grumbling about my sophistry, and he left with some sour mutterings.

I recognized that the setting of boundaries had become of particular importance. There was a confusion in his mind between intrusiveness and intimacy, public and private, action and communication. Hence he assumed that publishing the private poem to Ophelia was equivalent to my publishing his dreams. I had my first hints of the enclosed, claustrophobic form that his grandiosity could take, and how this fed on the delusion that he was acting for his real father rather than his usurping uncle. He saw his mission as correcting the distorted vision or values of his mother. The confusions adumbrated during these first few weeks dominated the first term of our brief period of analysis and came to a head eventually on the field of battle, which we were to call "the Mousetrap".

Meanwhile, as I took my customary lunchtime walk on the Heath the day of the "Batman" session, I meditated on certain failings of my own, which had begun, through Hamlet, to perco-late my consciousness. The weather was cold and blustery with scudding clouds, the beginning of the gales that would sweep the leaves from the trees, now still laden with autumn colour. I walked down the hill as far as the pond above South End Green and paused on the causeway across it, leaning on the rail, to watch the turbulence on the water. In the past, Beatrice had often used to come on these lunchtime walks, especially in the days when we lived in South End Green ourselves. Now she never did. We had moved up the hill to the affluent heart of Hampstead; but she had rented a share in a studio in Hackney and was rarely at home during the day. This was after she had accused me of ignoring her needs and undermining her by treating her as an ideal, a fiction of my own brain, rather than a person. At the time I could not imag-ine what she meant, so was sure she was wrong. I assumed she just needed to be released from the house, now that the girls could travel independently to school. But now, I could see that I was already developing an idealized view of Ophelia, on Hamlet's be-half; and I began to suspect that my over-romantic view of women was perhaps not something to be proud of but, on the contrary, was unconstructive, a type of self-indulgence. As though I implic-itly believed women could not be trusted to have unpleasant feelings. I wondered, as I walked back up the side of East Heath Road, if it was possible that Beatrice actually disliked me at times; and if so, when did it start?

* * *

As a result of these troubled musings, I told myself I must not be overprotective of Hamlet's relationship with Ophelia, or indeed with his parents. I must allow him to make his own discoveries, not contaminated by ideals of my own, which were themselves in turbulence. If only—in the months ahead—I had been able to heed my own advice! But I was overtaken by the rapidity of events.

The Prince

OPHELIA: He rais'd a sigh so piteous and profound
            As it did seem to shatter all his bulk
            And end his being. That done, he lets me go,
            And with his head over his shoulder turn'd
            He seem'd to find his way without his eyes,
            For out o'doors he went without their helps,
            And to the last bended their light on me.

                                              [II. i. 94–100]

"Looks like the old devil was right about women being untrustworthy and two-faced", were Hamlet's opening words at the next session. I realized, of course, that he was talking about the Ghost and Ophelia, and I wondered what had transpired over the weekend.

"The whole question is, which side expresses a woman's true nature—the inside or the outside", he said aggressively.

I thought this sounded ominous and asked him to explain.

"And I'm asking you—what the fuck is this thing called Beauty anyway?" he declaimed, gesticulating with his hands. I saw he was about to deliver a tirade. "Fools say, 'the world is so beautiful!' in their usual twittering plebspeak" (he mimicked a high idiotic whine). "What the hell does it really mean? Nothing—nothing at all. To mask the emptiness of their minds and their tightarsed suburban inhibitions, people go about labelling things as 'beautiful' just to show they're respectable and agree with each other. They all want to be part of the same mutual brainwashing system. That's all they need to give them a buzz. And it's exactly the same when it comes to women. Everyone is conditioned like Pavlov's dogs to start slavering at the sight of what is called a beautiful woman. But what is there really, underneath it all? Nothing but a pestilent congregation of vapours, a meaningless mess. A quintessence of dust. Right? But has anybody got the guts to admit it? Oh no, we're all supposed to keep up the show—keep it up, yeah, keep it up!"

He was fuming with sanctimonious rage. I suspected that much of this might be some sort of backlash from a sexual experience with Ophelia, about which he had said nothing so far. Even so I was surprised and somewhat incensed by this attack. I told Hamlet it was not the social conditioning of fashionable stereotypes that had aroused his violent ambivalence, but a subjective response which he felt was outside his control. He remained, therefore, firmly ensconced in his aggressive, macho "Batman" position.

He waited for me to finish my sentence but scarcely listened to what I was saying, and as soon as I drew breath he launched into the second half of his speech:

"And as for Truth—that's another social delusion, in fact a political one, even more pernicious. Professor Polly and his essay titles!" (So, I thought, is it an essay title that has put him in this rage?) "I can see him now", continued Hamlet, "walking backwards and forwards on the lecture platform, waving his arms in the pompous way he does when he's unloading his arthritic maxims. 'The truth', says he, wagging his finger in the air—'the truth is a direction which can only be found by indirections'! Ros and Gil were convulsed. Polly didn't notice—or if he did he'd have thought it was a sign of their youthful enthusiasm—following their worthy professor on the track of a 'truly scientific means of philosophical investigation of psychological structures!' So on he goes, 'hunting the trail of policy', as he calls it, and 'excavating the truth which is buried in the secret core of the mountain of evidence'. And all this crap delivered with such a naive, bright-eyed beaver look about him, as if he really believed he was on to some world-shaking discovery! Words, words, words!"

It was clear to me from all this, of course, that Hamlet's initial admiration for Professor Polack had switched suddenly to a virulent contempt, paralleling the switch in his attitude to his own father as indicated by the Ghost Dream. Stung by the suddenness and intensity of this attack and at a loss to explain it, I asked Hamlet whether the Professor had recently made any harsh criticisms of his academic work?

"God, no", replied Hamlet scathingly, "not Polly—nothing but mindless praise from him, even when I write an essay as lousy as the last one. I can tell it's lousy—he can't. He's a complete baby, his noises are meaningless. His last word of advice to us—believe it or not—was 'Brevity is the soul of wit'! As if he had any idea what brevity was! No, he's completely past it."

It was hard to assess to what extent Hamlet was exaggerating with his satirical treatment of the Professor. I remembered his parents' statement about Polack's high opinion of Hamlet's work. Possibly Hamlet was disappointed in his own estimation of it as a search for "truth". Clearly there was a connection between this "truth" and the hidden core of feminine beauty, which had enraged him as being disappointing or unattainable. I asked Hamlet if Polack had shown signs of disapproval over his interest in Ophelia?

"Why should he?" he said, surprised. "Anyway, Ophelia can twist him round her little finger."

So, as I suspected, the genesis of Hamlet's revulsion was to be found only within himself. I put it to him that once he was convinced of Polack's admiration for him, he decided the Professor must be an idiot—a "baby"—whom he had been fooling the whole time with his clever antics. He felt he had been leading the Professor round in "indirections". Not Ophelia, but he, had been twisting him round his finger. In effect he was accusing *himself* of being an impostor, and Polack of being a fool not to recognize it. He felt himself to be an intruder in this mysterious value-system of "truth and beauty". The problem still remained of whether he was an impostor in the sphere of his work, or Ophelia, or of both?

"Hang on", he objected, irritated, "now *you're* the one who's twisting! I was talking about how decrepit and unreliable Polly's judgement has become—his day is over. Mostly my essays are bloody good."

Nonetheless, I insisted, Polack's main folly—according to Hamlet—seemed to be to "believe in" Hamlet and his "truth". This was the gist of his account. He accused the Professor of misleading through "words, words, words". Yet, as we knew, Hamlet's own gift of the gab could be an equally unreliable vehicle for truth. The suggestion here was that he had been using words as a camouflage for "indirect" or intrusive entry into a world where he felt he had no place, no honest business.

"My whole point", protested Hamlet in aggrieved tones, "is that there *is no* truth—there is no such thing. It's an outdated concept, a form of brainwashing."

The "truth" we were talking about here, I said, was the sincerity of his feelings and motivation—in relation possibly to his work, certainly to Ophelia.

"So—what is it he really wants to know?" Hamlet finally exploded. "That I've been having it off with his precious daughter? So what—is that a 'truth'? It's no big deal, there's no mystery behind it. It's just that Polly likes to get his information through hints and circumlocutions. He has to make a baby-faced detective game out of it, an Easter-egg hunt. Unless it's wrapped up in a secret to start with, there's no satisfaction in the discovery."

Perhaps, I said, this particular mode of insincerity was one that applied to Hamlet himself. I pointed out that his method of informing me he had commenced sexual relations with Ophelia was itself a circuitous one.

"I didn't realize you were in such a hurry to know", he responded sarcastically.

His anxiety was, then, that he had used false or caricatural means to gain entry to Ophelia, holding her hostage before her father. Unable to tolerate the disturbing effect her beauty had on him, he had tried to capture or conquer it. In his hostage-holding technique there was, of course, an abuse of trust in relation to all involved.

"If anything, it's *me* who's the hostage in that set-up", said Hamlet. "She's her Daddy's girl, and I'm on probation."

Possibly, then, her beauty was aggravated in Hamlet's eyes by her closeness to her father. Unsure of his own position, he became suspicious that she was just her father's tool, a decoy used to betray his inmost "secrets" to the Professor. He felt trapped, essentially, by the confusing effect that beauty had on men's judgement.

"It's not her looks I'm suspicious about", said Hamlet; "it's the way she uses them—not just with me, with everybody."

Exactly, I confirmed. Her beauty was obvious to everybody; but the *meaning* of her beauty—that is, her feelings about Hamlet in particular—was not at all obvious. Hence his disturbance and frustration.

"I told you that myself", he said with disdain. "With women, the outside is no guide to the inside."

And now, I told him, he had found that sexual activity in itself was not the key to this mystery, not a magical solution. Possessing the beautiful object did not in itself lead to the truth—about either himself or Ophelia.

"You're really just an old-fashioned moralist, Dr Horacio, aren't you", he said. "I mean, there's nothing new in all this talk, is there? The beautiful object—the sacred cow."

His persistent scorn and irritation now began to make sense. His denigration of beauty, I said, was a way of denying the humiliation of an experience of impotence. The splitting of Ophelia into inside and outside, upper and lower parts of the body, paralleled his splitting of his father into good and bad, heroic and degenerate. By this means a degree of contempt for Ophelia had crept into his view of her; and this, I suggested, was in fact the cause of the impotence.

Hamlet shrugged this off, as he left the session, with a quiet, laconic cynicism. Something about this perturbed me even more than his raging. He clearly found the humiliation unbearable; and his glib sophistical slickness disguised, I could see, a deep failure of emotional contact. I suspected that Ophelia was becoming the new focus for his ambivalence—his love and his antagonism—superseding his parents and Polack. And his attacks on beauty and truth, which were now to be directed towards this vulnerable girl, wounded me deeply, so that I felt the urge to rise to her defence. The fighter-pilot stirred within me. Nevertheless I told myself, yet again, not to try to push the young couple together. Their relationship must evolve of itself.

One Monday morning a few sessions after this, Hamlet clomped down the steps in a filthy temper, bumping into walls and doorjambs with uncharacteristic clumsiness (normally he moved like a cat, quick and lithe). As he entered the room, he gave the carpet a vicious jab with the toe of his boot where it was slightly loose at the door junction, rucking it up.

"Why the hell can't you get this place fixed", he muttered; "it's the pits." He lay down with his hands still firmly ensconced in the pockets of his jacket, elbows sticking out, and announced:

"Well, Claude's chucked me out of the house at last."

(I was, as he knew, aware that his parents were in the process of moving out of their large house to a smaller flat, also in Hampstead—his father having decided to retire early from his business.) After an impressive pause filled with silent indignation, he complained:

"They've found themselves a place where there couldn't possibly be room for me. A bijou residence! I told Claude, of course—because I can't stand his way of secretly fiddling things behind my back—that I got the message completely. In fact, I was glad to have it out in the open."

I asked, did he not have a room of his own in the new flat?

"A room! A *room*", he snorted morosely. "Oh yeah—a room. I've been allocated a sort of cupboard half-way up the stairs, about the size of a hamster cage. And my mother babbles on about how they're going to have a skylight put in and fitted furniture and how it'll be 'ideal for me when I come home'. When I come home! They'll be lucky."

I pointed out the claustrophobic anxiety behind his sense of dispossession—enclosed and shut away by his parents in the "hamster cage", while "fiddling" was going on behind his back. It was reminiscent of the Ghost's complaint about weaning. There was also some envy of his parents' nest-building (which I related to the way he had scuffed my carpet); and a denial of his anxiety about why they needed to move—Claude's illness in particular.

"Nest-building!" he said contemptuously. "Behind my back— at their age—it's disgusting. Why do you think they chose the middle of the term to do it in, when I'm tied up at Cambridge? The fact is, the silly woman can't see through any of this—whatever Claude arranges, she raves over. Anything to keep him happy. That's a Pavlovian response for you. She's blinded by her own libido. So long as there's a place for their king-size double bed, and a sitting-room big enough for entertaining their legions of fascinating guests, everything is 'super duper'! According to *her*, it's going to be 'so much better, so much less to worry about'—all words Claude has put into her mouth, only she doesn't realize it, to disguise the fact that what he wants is to get me out the way."

This speech was delivered on a note of vitriolic outrage, and after a second's pause, Hamlet concluded: "No, I really can't stand Claude's style—it's suffocating. The bourgeois patriarch squatting at the centre of his web like some great fat spider. Quite honestly, I'm glad to quit."

This time, I connected Hamlet's fury and anxiety at being unhoused, thrown out, with the episode of impotence, which he had been too humiliated to confirm. This also was generated by his Batman identification with an aggressively patriarchal figure, ruler of women and the home, which made him feel "suffocated", imprisoned.

"Don't worry", said Hamlet, again ignoring my interpretation. "I'm taking steps to get out. I'm not one to bear a grudge, and I can see—our ways must part. I mean, there's no point sitting brooding like a constipated chicken, waiting for my uncle to change his spots. I can't live on air, promise-crammed. I need my freedom of interpretation. And now is my chance to catch the old goat at his own game, so everybody can see what's really going on. *Her*, in particular!"

The edge of excitement creeping into his voice was always an ominous sign—as was this talk about "freedom of interpretation" and "getting out", in the context of his enclosed, anxious state.

What, I asked him suspiciously, was "really going on" in his view?

"Well, the upshot is", he began with a certain triumph, "I've had it out with old Polly, and I'm going to be producing the Shakespeare play at the end of term. And when my mother sees it—hell, will it blow her mind! At last they'll see it how it really is! Even Claude's eyes might be opened—if he can blink in his brutish haze."

His zealous manner was giving me twinges of anxiety even before he confessed that whatever he had in mind was to be directed explicitly against his parents. Which play was it? I asked (for some reason, I was thinking of *Othello*).

"Believe it or not", he said, "it's *A Midsummer Night's Dream*. A surprising choice for me, you might think—a play for babies, really. But you'd be amazed at the dark and bestial fantasies there are hidden underneath all that fairy stuff. If you dig deep enough, you can really blow them at the moon!" Then he told me, with satisfaction, how Ophelia had agreed to be Titania and to perform a song-and-dance act from *Cabaret*, which he had inserted; though her brother had refused to act the part of one of her attendants: "I tried to explain that in *my* Dream, which for Christ's sake is a Dream of 1973, I don't need fairies who are little ballet-girls, I need big hulking men, and he'd have been perfect. What the hell—I've got Rosenfeld and Gildstein down instead for Peaseblossom and Cobweb, and a couple of first years—Peacock and Seaman—for Moth and Mustardseed. They're all going to double as the mechanicals, to bring out the ambiguity of the whole thing. I'm going to do Bottom myself, of course. That's the basic set-up already. The art, you see, lies in getting the right people teamed up to express my message."

As I listened to his "basic set-up", anger was rising in me. He was converting the play into some sort of omnipotent masturbatory phantasy founded on "big hulking" mechanical-fairy-fingers. Now it was Shakespeare's turn to be held hostage. But that in itself was the least of my worries. I was disturbed by the mixture of sanctimony and violence in his language—such as "blowing at the moon" and "blowing his mother's mind"; and even more, by the public acting-out of this phantasy with himself and Ophelia in fixed positions at the centre of it all. In explaining this to Hamlet, I warned him of the possibility of damaging his private relationship with this girl.

"She's *my* girlfriend!" he protested, not so much possessively as authoritatively, in the manner of a young eighteenth-century aristocrat talking about his housemaid. I said that did not entitle him to treat her as his whore.

He laughed unpleasantly, a little surprised, and defended himself by saying: "I credited you with being more enlightened about the whole scene of sexual freedom. A radical staging like mine is bound to shock the older generation—some of them. You're obviously cramped by the same old-fashioned values as the rest."

Slogans such as "sexual freedom" and "freedom of interpretation", I said, were banners for action and would contaminate his private relationships. It was the omnipotent "fuck, fuck" side of himself taking over again.

"What's the difference anyway between what you call my 'slogans' (just because you don't like them) and your 'values', which are simply out of date (but I don't hold that against you)?" he demanded.

Values were flexible, I explained—they were a basis for communication between people. Slogans were for imposing his will on people.

"Honour thy father and mother ... is what it boils down to, isn't it, according to you?" he sneered, as if even I must consider this "value" too degradingly simplistic, a *reductio ad absurdum*.

All right, I said with some impatience, he could consider "honouring Shakespeare" as a reasonable starting-point for his play production, and move on from there, instead of arranging everything and everybody around his own directorial role, to "express his message" as he put it. Shakespeare was, after all, the father of his own play, and the play had its own aesthetic dignity, not to be violated.

"Ah! so that's it after all!" he said in a tone of triumph, as if he had winkled the secret of my resistance out of me. "You just can't stomach my interpretation. I knew it! All this charade about psychoanalysis being a scientific process—now it turns out you're just a literary romantic after all. To you Shakespeare is some sort of god, not to be profaned by the realities of everyday life—you can't see he's simply one of the great hacks, churning out plays for his patrons!"

And to my gloom and frustration, he left with his princely omnipotence not merely intact but inflamed. I saw that I had failed utterly to deflate it. And for a while after this, Hamlet seemed careful not to say too much about the play, although I was aware of it fulminating in the background. He clearly didn't want any interference and developed a subtly condescending attitude to me, as if it were up to me to re-establish my status as his professional confidante after exceeding my brief. Correspondingly, he was meticulous about punctuality and other formal aspects of the analytic setting, but in a way that suggested this was really a substitute for true cooperation, a pretence to disguise his essential secretiveness. Moreover, I could see that I, too, had become a hostage to his princely antics, now that he had—inevitably—discovered my own aesthetic values; and in this context it made me feel strangely vulnerable. I counselled myself to be more cautious for the time being and to wait for dreams. Hamlet was having difficulty remembering these, but eventually he did bring me an interesting and thoughtful dream, which, despite its air of egocentricity, seemed to augur hopefully for his relationship with Ophelia. I began to believe this might escape damage from the play after all.

This dream, which we came to call the "To be or not to be" Dream because it was about the question of "being" a lover, went as follows:

> "Doctor Horacio, I do not know
> Whether to fall in love, or not to fall
> In love. Sick with indecision,
> The current of my resolution's gone
> Awry. Was this the drink my father drank
> That shot him into a sky of troubles?—to taste
> The heartache and the thousand natural shocks
> That strike like lightning from the heart of life's
> Outrageous stormclouds, whose consummation
> Is only death. What dream can help me now,
> The ignorant survivor of his catastrophe?

Suppose I shuffle off this mortal coil,
My naked newborn soul can only pause
In apprehension, puzzled as it stands
On the cliff's brink, while all before, the world
Spreads out into the misty distance. Why fly
To sins as yet unknown—and should I jump,
Or fall? And even as I stand and think,
Her shaping spirit awakes my recollection
Like a chill vapour of early dawn, and I pray
That love and fame to nothingness will sink."

"I know what the dream means", stated Hamlet with quiet confidence. "It means I really am in love with Ophelia after all. I was thinking that yesterday after the rehearsal. Rosenfeld said I was lucky to be going out with Ophelia, he wouldn't mind her himself—he was quite offhand, sort of joky, and walked straight off. But it made me think, yes, it was only natural everybody should want Ophelia. I really *was* lucky. And a sort of warm glow went through me—I felt strange, and sad. I thought maybe we could really make it together."

Then he began to talk about the dream, and how "all that about consummation meant sex, not death" and was about the sensuality in his family, which he'd "inherited but could accept better now", because he knew that Ophelia really understood him—even his hang-ups. After all, they'd worked together on the play, and she really understood what he wanted her to do, and it was a fact that she was "fabulous—everybody said so".

"It's Coleridge, you know, about 'shaping spirit'," he informed me. "And that about love and fame is Keats—we've been doing them this term. I used to think, who wants Romantic wish-wash about moons and waterfalls when you could have compasses and telescopes like the Metaphysicals—which is so much more like real life. But now I see I can use them after all!"

I noted the childish egocentricity that Hamlet's confidences in me still had, when he felt I was somehow "pleased" with him. It was an indication of his instability; he could easily swing back into manic arrogance. His enthusiasm for both Ophelia and the Romantic poets seemed to be grounded to some degree in the way in which he could "use" them in projects of his own. He still did not have the concept of communicating with his girlfriend, or of learning from the poets. He believed Ophelia "understood" him; I tried tactfully to suggest, had he ever considered whether he understood *her*? Similarly, he made judgements about the usefulness of poetic diction in "real life" (meaning, to him) without first considering whether he had understood the poets' usage.

This lack of humility was very characteristic of what I described to him as his "princely" mentality. It was, of course, directed towards me too: I was a member of his entourage, allotted a strictly limited function of observing and recording, receiving his confidences, but not allowed to curb his acting-out. That would be going too far—a type of indecorum. Thus he had fixed on Shakespeare's *Dream* and, pre-empting my role as interpreter of dreams, he handed over his own version to me as his amanuensis or scribe. I pointed out to him that he was treating me as his future biographer, witness to the facts of his emotional display, while paralysing any effective intervention on my part. At this he laughed indulgently, taking it—from his prince's viewpoint—as a compliment to his management. Once again, I was the one left feeling hurt and vulnerable.

I returned, therefore, to the interpretation of his latest dream—which was, like all his dreams, full of emotional significance. I emphasized its importance first of all as a pause for thought, which was both rare and welcome. Acting-out (the "current of resolution") was suspended in mid-air, allowing a breathing-space. At that moment nothing was inevitable. The ready-made channels down which action was supposed to plunge became "puzzled" (to use the dream's very evocative word). Hamlet's direction was no longer obvious, no longer propelled by slogans and sanctimony.

This meant also, however, that his position regarding "falling in love" was a tenuous and unresolved one. The picture in the dream was not quite the same as the "warm glow" he had described himself, a glow of satisfaction and possession, the triumph of having secured a desirable girl. The dream showed that in fact things were much more complicated. Here, love was associated with "shocks", "heartache", lightning, and so on, and the implication was that his father seemed to have been prepared to face this emotional turbulence. It was an interesting variation on the theme of his father's heroism in the Ghost Dream. Hamlet himself was maybe "on the brink" of such an experience, but he had not actually "jumped" as yet. His tentative "puzzlement" suggested a certain disappointment in his sense of gratifying Ophelia and in his own sexual gratification, which was not as immediate or over-whelming as he had expected. I pointed out to Hamlet that he was still very much a beginner in sexual love and was only gradually discovering the complications and confusions that were involved in becoming a lover.

It was, indeed, a very sensitive and revealing dream. Poten-tially it could be a great help to Hamlet in his relationship with his girlfriend. In my enthusiasm for the dream, however, I had over-estimated Hamlet's capacity to tolerate any interpretation that seemed to him to undermine his princely dignity. Making the con-nection with the Ghost Dream, and reminding Hamlet that in this area his stature was still as it were lower than his father's, nearly lost me my tenuous role as confidante.

"You wait till you see my play", he said coldly. "It puts all these chivalric hangups about love in a modern perspective. Claude and his type will be utterly deflated." (Was I, I wondered, now one of "his type"?) "You are coming to see it, aren't you?" he added suddenly, alarmed. I explained that I did not think it advisable.

"You'll miss something", he said meaningfully.

I didn't doubt it. In fact, I could barely tolerate even the thought of his arrogant desecration of the play, though my curios-ity to see Ophelia almost tempted me to consider creeping in secretly. This was, however, too risky and was overridden by my anxiety over the boost I knew it would give to Hamlet's omnipo-tence, should he find out. In addition to this, I felt the play was wasting analytic time, providing an outlet for Hamlet's directorial or princely antics, without allowing us really to get our teeth into these in the analytic context. Whenever we came across evidence of his omnipotence or egocentricity, he would automatically take shelter in the Play, as if this would provide the answer to every-thing. Anybody who saw his play—it was implied—would lose their old-fashioned inhibitions and receive enlightenment. The New Prince would come into his own.

This time, as Hamlet passed me on his way out of the consult-ing-room, he looked momentarily but intensely into my eyes and said, "You'll see, Dr Horacio, there are more things in heaven and earth than in your 'dreaming' philosophy. Bye for now." His dark smouldering glance, under the strips of lanky dark hair falling vertically over his cheeks, gave me a sense of extreme foreboding. I told myself to prepare for some volcanic eruption in his state of mind.

The Mousetrap

OPHELIA: You are as good as a chorus, my lord.
HAMLET: I could interpret between you and your love if I could see
           the puppets dallying.
OPHELIA: You are keen, my lord, you are keen.
HAMLET: It would cost you a groaning to take off my edge.
OPHELIA: Still better, and worse.
HAMLET: So you mistake your husbands.—Begin, murderer. Leave
           thy damnable faces and begin. Come, the croaking raven
           doth bellow for revenge.

                                                    [III. ii. 240–248]

I t was Hamlet himself who first described his version of Shakespeare's *Midsummer Night's Dream* as a "mousetrap" intended
to exhibit to his parents the stupid and pornographic nature
of their lovemaking. (It transpired that in fact Claude was in the
habit of calling Gertrude his "mouse".) By the end of this play
production, however, every member of our little drama had sus-
tained some degree of insult or injury.

"There's a political message here", he explained to me, during one of his compulsive lectures, when I had to exercise all my energy and ingenuity to get a word in edgewise. "You could say I'm a man with a mission. I need a play that I can take off in—and to take shape, the play needs me. That's the wonderful thing about poetry. It cries out to be rewritten by succeeding generations. Now that notions of authorial Authority have been discredited, new poets like me are faced with the public duty of altering the old bard's canon to suit ourselves. That—of course—is the challenge. People should thank their lucky stars there's someone like me around who can strip the tinsel wrapping off this play and expose the secret bestiality of the affair. You've got to be cruel to be kind."

These were terrorist tactics, I told him, with their characteristic mixture of sanctimony and complacency. I had tried repeatedly to warn Hamlet of the danger of taking "revenge" on his objects through manic enactments. His talk of being a "man with a mission" and "taking off" in the play demonstrated acting-out on the lines of the Batman Dream—the aggressive aspect of the Ghost–pilot. In the Ghost Dream he had been so confused with his father's penis that he could not distinguish whether it was heroic or assaultive. Now he was acting as though he were living inside it, taking military action on what he had called this "play for babies". The play was Shakespeare's baby, and he was holding it hostage in order to attack his parents.

"You sound like Polly, with your worshipful phraseology", he said, evidently trying to restrain the contempt in his voice and speaking as though to a rather slow-witted child. "This isn't the classroom, it's the stage. It's worship that results in the death of art. Until I give this play an audience and make it relevant to the complex issues of today, it's going to stay stuffed in the attic of English Heritage, to be guarded by fossils like Professor Polly!"

And so, for many sessions, I made fruitless attempts to penetrate the sanctimony of what he called his "mission" and put him back in touch with the ambivalence and hostility towards the aesthetic that had come out clearly in his tirades against "truth" and "beauty". Whenever I made any headway with this, he became irritable and contemptuous and put me in my place; then—probably at the next session—he would be furtive and a little anxious, surreptitiously seeking reassurance that he hadn't in fact made an enemy of me. But the actual content of what he called my "sermonizing" slipped over him like water off a duck's back. I reflected on the particular difficulty I had with Hamlet in describing the transference without the help of dreams. Unless a dream was in front of us, with its graphic evidence for the transference, it was easy to be seduced into the conflictual debating mode that he invited, and then the emotionality of our relationship was dissipated.

To one of those "furtive" sessions, at last, he brought an odd little dream *about a huge old yew tree growing in an enclosure, with steps and a stone balustrade in front and a stately building in the background (reminding him of the Fitzwilliam Museum). From inside the tree came a strange wailing voice, crying urgently at regular intervals, "Set me free, set me free!" At last the warden came along, unlocked the gate into the enclosure, and tapped the tree with his stick, upon which a small creature like a squirrel emerged from an opening in the bark and darted quickly away. But then the warden appeared distraught and ran round the tree in circles, crying "My money, my daughter! My money, my daughter!"* In the dream this had not seemed comical, but a logical way of addressing some serious problem.

Hamlet told me that the tree with steps and the stately façade resembled the stage-set for his play, and that the warden, who was bald with a pointed beard, reminded him of Professor Polack. I could see that the dream had something to do with his claustrophobia and with the release of trapped femininity, but it was hard to say whether the Professor–warden was the imprisoner, or the liberator, or both. Hamlet had not long ago described him sarcastically as a "guardian" of literature; hence the association with the Museum; but this also suggested an uncreative, sterile guardianship, perhaps linked with the idea of "money" more than of "daughter". The warden's words about his money and his daughter also took us back to the "Chocolate-Box" Dream at the beginning of his analysis, in which the Professor had exhorted his children to "grow and prosper". In that dream there was a similar ambiguity about the idea of prosperity—did this mean growth and development, or did it mean wealth and success?

"That's Polly all right", said Hamlet sarcastically. "It's hard to tell which is his greater obsession—whether he owns Shakespeare or Ophelia." And he admitted that he had had an altercation with the Professor after he had come to see the dress rehearsal of his play. "Well, what can you expect at his age?" he shrugged, with casual disdain. "His opinions are all fuddled up—he liked this, but then he didn't like that, and then again . . . blah blah."

I interpreted that it was me, not just Polack, whom he was attacking for having a proprietary attitude towards both the play and Ophelia. I was also, of course, the guardian of psychoanalysis. The dream confirmed the location of our current problem in the realm of aesthetic vitality, and the need for the aesthetic object to have its freedom. This was our constant theme in the context of the Play as an aesthetic, feminine object, in which resided Hamlet's own femininity—linked also with his relation to Ophelia.

At this, Hamlet turned his head and said aggressively, raising his hand in an oratorical gesture, "The fact is, Dr Horacio, you've got such fixed notions about this fucking play, that in spite of going on about it incessantly, you can't even be bothered to come and see my production!"

I explained again that it would be inappropriate for me to come and see it—it was better for him to talk to me about it. With a play, he retorted, "everything was in the context and the staging"—my enslavement to the domination of words was as bad as Polly's: "If you actually came to see it—especially the way Ophelia does it—you'd be knocked out!"

Describe it, I told him—reproaching myself for my cowardice in having hoped it might blow over without my having to hear too much about it.

"All right", he began, with defiance and a certain pomposity. "You have to realize, to start off with, that the core of the whole thing is the scenes between Bottom and Titania in the wood, and the wood, of course, is the façade for a brothel, a high-class bordello, and it's the place where all these Athenian aristocrats go to learn about sex and how to do it—that's why they can't get married till they've been there. Snakes with double tongues and enamelled skin, thickets and bushes of pubic hair, streakings of magic juice—it's all code for sexual parts. The fairies are there for the foreplay, to oil the process and get it all working—sucking out the honey-bags, lighting their thighs with glow-worms . . . I mean, you've only got to look at those names—Squash, Peascod,

Mustardseed. Titania calls it "doing courtesies". So the fairies are all sexual aids—that's why I've got them doubling with the mechanicals; they're dressed up in rugby gear and they do a brilliant song-and-dance routine with Titania, a kind of classy strip act—you ought to see it, I mean really. When Bottom comes along, it's all jazzed up, because the fairies are in *his* service then, so he can use them to service Titania. Titania, you see, is still a virgin, and that's why she's pissed off with Oberon—he's impotent (which explains why he's so obsessed with the drugs scene). But once she's found a real man, who wears his balls on his head (his arse-head, of course) she closes her trap on him, and like he says, he hasn't got 'wit enough to get out of this wood'—he's stuck between her legs with his "tongue tied up", that is, his prick. He doesn't mind, of course—that's his forte. And *she* doesn't care if he's some stupid labourer—that's all the better, in fact she wants to enslave herself to him:

"I will purge thy mortal grossness so,
That thou shalt like an airy spirit go"

she says to Bottom—that's code for the male orgasm, of course, 'purging'. Then there's her coy moan about the moon's 'watery eye', which makes 'every little flower' weep (and it's obvious what that means), 'lamenting some enforced chastity'. The fact is, of course, she's dying to have her chastity enforced, and that's what Bottom does for her—

"So doth the woodbine the sweet honeysuckle
Gently entwist; the female ivy so
Enrings the barky fingers of the elm."

Fingers or prick—so long as it's twisting up her she'll ring her muscles round it, and there you have the female orgasm! So long as it's 'barky' she's happy . . . that's Shakespearean ambiguity for you"—he finished in a triumphant and provocative manner.

And, indeed, I found I was provoked—intolerably. It was now crystal clear that what had started as an act of "revenge" on his parents, trying to split them through ridiculing their sexuality, had switched its focus like a spotlight onto Ophelia. She was now the primary victim of his abusive phantasy, and all the macho obscenity of his interpretation of the play was directed at her,

holding her up in the eyes of everyone as his whore. I didn't
need to see the play, I said, to realize from his description that
his antagonism was also directed at the analysis, displaying for
ridicule the world of "the dream" and my role as the dream-
interpreter.

"Oh, God—this really is too boring, Dr Horacio", was his deri-
sive response to my anxieties. "I can't understand why it bugs you
so much. Whose reputation is it you're worrying about anyway?
It's me, not you, who's on the line. As for Ophelia—she *wants* to
be in it, I'm not forcing her. It's the ideal vehicle for her talents."

I told him he was completely oblivious to the contempt he
was displaying for Ophelia, presenting her as slave to his sexual
manipulations. It was the same as making Shakespeare's play
the victim of his directorial twistings—the "indirections" of the
intruder, ensconced in this identification with an aggressive
"princely" penis. This was not "Shakespearean ambiguity", but an
imposition of his own—a "mousetrap" in which everyone was
caught—his parents, his girlfriend, Shakespeare, and the analysis
itself.

He swore agitatedly and said, "At last I've got the chance to
do something really creative, and all you lot can do is shit on
it! Well—all I can say is, dirtymindedness is in the eye of the
beholder!"

And he departed in high dudgeon, looking daggers at me.

Shortly after this, the play production was over, and now the
Christmas break was approaching. Hamlet appeared at the last
Saturday session with a manic, self-righteous gleam in his eyes.
He was wearing a huge, heavy chain over his jacket, which gave
him the appearance of the Lord Mayor. He hardly glanced at me
as he strode in with tight-set lips, flung himself on the couch, and
commenced one of his tirades.

"Believe it or not, Her Royal Highness summoned me last
night to an exclusive interview in her private apartments. Naturally I was most gratified, given my humble status as the household
cat, to be vouchsafed this rare and privileged opportunity for a few
intimate words alone with my mother. After all, she never noticed
my existence when we actually lived together (*much* too busy for
that)—though she's obviously found plenty of time to jabber to old
Polly and the rest of her retinue *about* me! As for High and Mighty

himself—he was skulking somewhere out of sight, as he always does when there's anything unpleasant going on. So much for his patriarchal guts."

Hamlet then explained that he had gone to his parents' flat after his last session, not intending to stay the night, but to pick up some things to take to Nando's and to get something to eat "because there's never any grub at *his* place". His parents, he knew, were out with friends, watching "some slushy Bergman film" at the Everyman. But as he was about to leave, his mother had returned, alone "or pretending to be", and insisted on speaking to him.

"'Hamlet, my dear', she begins" (he began), "'I have been wanting to speak to you for a while' (well, who's been stopping you?), 'but it's been hard to know how to approach the subject—you've been so much leading your own life lately' (yes I have had a bit on my mind—moving my gear into Forte and Nando's for a start, 'cos I can't stand the Bijou Residence any longer even for the vac—). Then she whines, in her nauseating, faltering female way: 'These have, of course, been rather difficult times for all of us' (oh yeah?) 'and it is imperative to pay some serious thought to it' (good, good—very glad, I'm all in favour of serious thought—can she possibly have noticed there is more to life than fornication?). Next, I have to listen to how she, and Claude, and Polly, have all been 'worrying' about my behaviour (that is, gossiping about me behind my back—thank you, dear Mother, I am most flattered to be the object of your dedicated attention, so much in demand by all and sundry—Sundry in particular). And, finally, she draws herself up to her full height of five foot three and makes the magisterial pronouncement:

"'My dear Hamlet, we really must discuss what is to be done—you are no longer a child, and neither is she.'"

(Ah! I thought, with some foreboding—now we are getting there.) He continued, however, with his circuitous rant:

"Then off again into all this twaddle about serious intentions and feminine feelings and other wish-wash that I suppose she gets from films and novels—such is the insatiable appetite of the female sex for sentimental slurp! They make me mad. I tried to get it across to her that *my* feelings were real ones—doubtless beyond her comprehension—and that the subtleties of my mind had their existential profundity in what was quite simply space-aeons away from TV serials and Bergman mopies."

Here Hamlet paused for a moment to let the injured self-right-eousness of his declaration sink into my consciousness. Now, I thought, he is finally going to tell me. Well? I asked.

"And then, only then—" he declared solemnly, "after all this bullshit, does she finally say to me: 'Perhaps you don't realize that Ophelia is pregnant?'"

Oh, God, I thought.

"That was how she said it, the cow—all smug and quiet, and with no warning at all—just to make a complete fool of me! I could have hit her. I felt as though she'd hit *me*. I don't think I did hit her, I can't quite remember—perhaps I shook her by the shoulders or something, I felt sick with rage—literally, I thought I was going to vomit. I just remember rushing out and slamming the door."

I was dismayed at this unexpected blow, coming upon us at the worst possible time in the analysis. When sorrows come, I thought to myself, it's not as single spies, but in battalions. Hamlet's mur-derous feelings were not being contained within the analytic context but were erupting outside it, and yet he seemed oblivious of the implications of his violence. I realized (though he didn't) that Gertrude had been frightened of him, and with good reason. It was essential to bring him out of his sanctimonious cocoon and back into emotional contact. I warned Hamlet more emphatically than ever of the dangers of allowing himself to be taken over by the assaultive, anti-feminine masculinity of the Batman Dream, and how this had very nearly resulted in actual violence against his mother.

He listened to my urgent interpretation with irritable impa-tience, and accused me of being seduced by his mother "like all the rest":

"You just can't see, can you", he said sourly, "that it's me who's the victim in all this, not my blasted mother. Do you sup-pose I was going to murder her, like some Gothic heroine? I'm entitled to my feelings too, you know! What do you think I am, a poker-faced cold fish like Forte or somebody?" (Forte, it appeared, being a friend of Nando's to whom Hamlet had taken a particular dislike.) Then he continued, more savagely: "And it's *her* fault as

much as anyone's—yes, Ophelia's! another favourite of yours—
she who in her beauty and innocence can do no wrong—unless, of
course, corrupted by some worthless and depraved specimen such
as myself—Why couldn't she tell me first? Instead, she runs
straight to her father—the doddering old idiot—and *he* flaps off to
my mother, and then all three of them gang up against me behind
my back, gloating that now they've really got something they can
hold against me. Maybe they can tie me down for good in the
straitjacket of bourgeois matrimony, so that I can be a pompous
prat like the rest of them—'Now Hamlet, be a good boy!'—and
she's the one who put me straight in their trap!"

He finished with an outraged flourish, which nevertheless concealed a new note of insistent anxiety. I pointed out that Ophelia
would have found it impossible to communicate anything to him
about the pregnancy in his present paranoid state. And it was not
parental expectations that disturbed him, but hopes and fears of
his own. As in the "To be or not to be" Dream, what frightened
him was the idea of falling in love, entering a state of hopeful-
ness—the possibility that he, too, could be a real lover. All the
victims of his present comprehensive attack represented his own
love-objects—his mother, Ophelia, myself in the analysis, Shakespeare. These love-objects evoked in him expectations of himself.

At this he swore and hit his fist on the edge of the couch, to
express his unutterable ridicule and rage. Then he hissed, "Can't
you put yourself in *my* position for once—can't you even *see* how
they're all ganging up to attack *me*?"

I said he was so convinced he was the victim that it was difficult for him to see that it was something in himself which he was
attacking—the internal objects, which represented the kind of
beauty that was truth. Truthful communication with such an internal object, through his external love-objects, would involve
sacrificing his vanity and egoism. He could conceive of trying to
control Ophelia, and of Ophelia trying to control him, but not of
engaging his development with hers on a level deeper than the
possession of physical beauty. This would be to discover the inner
beauty or truth of a person, the love-object. He could not conceive
that his parents had done this, that Shakespeare had done it with
his play, that I did it with psychoanalysis—that this is what is
meant by being a lover.

"You're always on the woman's side, aren't you?" he said accusingly, "whatever the facts of the case—they're always right, and I'm always wrong!"

And what, I asked, *were* the facts of the case? To what extent was it an accident, and to what extent did he really believe Ophelia was "innocent" and he was responsible? (For, surprised though I had been by the news of Ophelia's pregnancy, Hamlet's persistent hostility to the event gave me the increasing impression that it was not the "accident" it had first seemed.)

"The facts", he said irritably and evasively, "are that Ophelia's as old as I am and this is 1974—are you accusing me of rape or something? Because I can assure you, nothing could be further from the 'truth'—as you like to have it. Like all women, she knows precisely what she's doing, and she's been doing it with God knows how many others besides me!"

I reminded him of the aristocracy of Athens who had to go to whores to practise sex because they were frightened of impotence. He himself was acting like one of those aristocrats.

"Why the hell should I believe it was anything to do with me anyway?" he then exploded. "There's nothing to prove it was me. You should hear what Nando says about her—he knows her better than most. And I told you about Rosenfeld—he's a sly bugger! What about Forte? He's been after her for ages—he was always snooping about in the wings during the performance—you could see for a fact he was just waiting to grab Ophelia after the show!"

This, I said immediately, was his jealousy. Previously, in his princely omnipotence, he had assumed Ophelia was his indisputable possession. Now, it suddenly seemed to him that she was surrounded by men waiting to seize her from the wings. The fact of her pregnancy had jolted him out of his security, his arrogance.

"Jealous! I'm not jealous of *Forte*!" he sneered.—"And you're wrong, I don't think I own her—it's her business. There's no accounting for taste. I don't pretend to be her keeper—I mean, half the nights of the week I'm down here seeing you! I just think she should honestly admit who did it, that's all."

Evidently the pregnancy was something inconceivable to him, an event that could not possibly have been generated by their relationship. He really couldn't believe it had anything to do with him, though I still suspected he had engineered it in order to confirm his ownership of Ophelia, but then found himself completely thrown by the reality. Instead of securing his position as the prince, it made him feel yet again that he had been ejected, humiliated—somebody else must have done it behind his back. I pondered on this with interest, and much more sympathy, as his youthful vulnerability (so long obscured by the Mousetrap) presented itself to me with renewed force. My anger evaporated a little as I considered the likely doubts about his own success as a lover that lay behind his new experience of jealousy. His activities as a lover, he felt, seemed to bear no relation to this pregnancy which had struck like a bolt from the blue.

Meanwhile, I wondered, who or what was this "Forte" who had suddenly appeared within the circle of his intimate acquaintance? Whoever he might refer to in actuality, I could see that I was going to have a long and hard struggle with what one might call Hamlet's own "Forte" consciousness. This was his hardening omnipotence—his defence against his new vulnerability.

To the final session before the break, however, he brought a dream that marked a watershed in the analysis.

The dream referred to the last performance of his play, which his parents had come to watch.

In the dream, *his mother was sitting in the front row, watching the play. Then she got up and began to walk slowly and deliberately up on to the stage where he was. She was wearing long voluminous robes and had a diadem on her forehead. The heavy crimson stage curtains closed behind her, and she spoke reproachfully to Hamlet, saying:*

"Hamlet, you have greatly offended your father, and he is no longer prepared to play on the same stage with you."

Hamlet replied, "Don't you like this mirror image of your inmost parts?" Then he noticed a strange twitching movement low down amongst the folds of her dress, which he found repulsive, and he instinctively stabbed at it viciously with a stage dagger—to discover that it was not an animal, as he had supposed, but Professor Polack, the size of a dwarf, bowing and grinning. His mother gave a deep sigh and sank to her knees, saying, "Hamlet, you have broken my heart in two." Then the dwarf Professor grew in stature like one of those genii from a magic lamp and metamorphosed into his father, Claude, who seemed to hover over

him. His father was clothed in a familiar loose Japanese-style silk dress-
ing gown with a water-lily pattern, whose sleeves moved as if in a light
breeze as he held out his arms towards Hamlet, saying:

> *"Remember, Hamlet, taint not thy mind nor harm thy*
> *mother."*

Hamlet felt beads of sweat on his forehead. He felt he was looking at a
ghost. What seemed to terrify him specifically was his father's gaze fixed
on him. In fact, he begged this new Ghost:

> *"Do not look on me, lest you convert*
> *The blood-red colour of my masculine revenge*
> *Into watery tears and the sort of giving way*
> *That would trouble a woman."*

Then the stage curtains opened again, and Hamlet, to his humiliation,
saw the cartoon-like faces of the audience leering and laughing.

Here was the "Mousetrap" indeed, and Hamlet's own dream-
analysis of the significance of the acting-out of the past many
weeks. At last I had some clear evidence to show Hamlet his little-
boy vulnerability, as he managed to relinquish the claustrophobic
identification with a macho internal father which had been domi-
nating his state of mind.

His difficulty in relating the dream was evident. In sarcastic
tones he mimicked a high plaintive voice for his mother and a
deep ponderous one for his father. It seemed to be the final "humiliation" that rankled, rather than the murderous implications of
his own actions in the dream.

"I'm sick of being treated like a child!" he fumed. "One minute
they pat me on the head and the next they kick me up the arse."

In the dream, I agreed, he was indeed a child, who had intruded into his parents' bedroom (represented by the stage),
acting as if he owned the place. Indeed, the double layers of dra-
pery (the long dress, the curtains closing behind her) indicated his
mother's "inmost parts", which he had attacked by stabbing the
dwarf-size Professor–baby within her.

"Silly old prick", snapped Hamlet. "The voice of moralism getting its just deserts."

I reminded him of how he had been driven out of his little
room, the "hamster cage", owing to his claustrophobic sense of

being inside his mother, controlling her. This had also been his attitude to Ophelia, directing her in the "Mousetrap". Her pregnancy, however, had undermined this role. And now the linking of his various father-figures to warn him against damaging his internal objects suggested that there could be a transforming, reparative power at work, very different from the punitive "revenge" of a disciplinarian father or the disordered thinking of a word-twisting father.

"You mean, it's as though they're all ganging up against me", was Hamlet's paranoid response. "I don't need a Ghost in a dream to tell me that."

It was, I said, his own continual splitting that was being confronted by the dream—like his mother saying her heart was "split in two".

"That's your interpretation, anyway", he muttered. From *my* point of view it would be a good thing if she learned to make distinctions."

He didn't like to think the idealized fighter-pilot, the sensual diplomat–businessman, the "guardian" of literature, and indeed myself as the protector of psychoanalysis could all be aspects of the same internal father-figure.

"Oh yeah—come on!" he sneered. "you put stuff like that in your scientific papers, so-called! Yet you object to poetic ambiguities in my interpretation of a play."

It was the dream itself that disturbed him, I said, not my interpretation of it—the emotional facts were there in front of us.

I was disturbed myself by his present instability, and I emphasized to him the warning of violence contained in the dream, and the aggressive feelings aroused by Ophelia's pregnancy. It was impossible to tell what form his vulnerability and sense of humiliation might take during the two-week break in analysis. Nevertheless the dream was clearly a turning-point in terms of Hamlet's release from his claustrophobic identification with his father's overtly military hero–penis. This marked the beginning of the end of his delusory "uncle–father". I pointed out the reparative direction indicated by the new Ghost–father when he said that revenge on womanly feelings could be converted into "tears". On this tenuous contact I had to base my hopes that he would survive the Christmas break without erupting or collapsing.

The Grave

HAMLET: Witness this army of such mass and charge,
Led by a delicate and tender prince,
Whose spirit, with divine ambition puff'd,
Makes mouths at the invisible event,
Exposing what is mortal and unsure
To all that fortune, death, and danger dare,
Even for an eggshell.

[IV. iv. 47–53]

The Monday after the Christmas break, Hamlet was delivered to the door in an MG sports car, twenty minutes late for the early morning session. He stumbled uncertainly down the steps and entered the consulting-room looking uncharacteristically dirty and dishevelled, his clothes smelling strongly of stale tobacco smoke and marijuana.

"Sorry I'm late, old man", he began; "couldn't make it any earlier. If it hadn't been for Forte I wouldn't have made it at all. The fact is, I don't feel too brill. I know what you're thinking—

you're surprised at me having anything to do with him, seeing he's such a pansy joker. Well—it's sheer coincidence. He just gave me a lift, that's all—on the way to his office. I had a long way to come. He's cool enough in his way—got an MG Coupe. The fact is, I had the most awful dream last night—or the night before. We were all at this groovy affair at Forte's place in the country—his mother's place that is. Bedfordshire. Some of us are still there. Amazing."

It was the first time I had seen Hamlet befuddled through drink or drugs (of which he was normally very contemptuous, claiming he didn't need to indulge in such stuff, and satirizing the "moronic glazed" attitudes of his friends when "stoned"). But I wondered if this was all that lay behind his disjointed attention and inquired after the dream he had mentioned.

"Yeah, that was pretty awful . . ." he drawled. "They've got a house right out in the country, with a huge barn, where everybody could doss down together. You could really freak out—there was live music all night—two groups, lights, a proper bar. All professional stuff, nothing tatty or amateur."

I pointed out that he had been so impressed by the facilities at this party that he had failed to keep his commitment to me.

"Look, man, I said I was sorry, didn't I?" he said more energetically, recovering his powers of speech. "I knew you'd be ratty, but it couldn't be helped. Everybody was there, everybody. Weird, really, I always thought Forte was poncy and stuck-up, but now I reckon he's just shy. And lonely. He's an only child, like me—but spoilt to death. He's always had everything he wants— this was his twenty-first birthday party. His people are pretty interesting too. His father is away most of the time, he does documentaries and things. But his mother is amazing, really way out, I've never come across a woman like her, with such a powerful personality. She writes articles on progressive culture—you know—self-awareness, alternative society and stuff. She's Lifestyle Editor on *The Dictator*" (he said impressively). "So it's her business to see what's coming before anyone else does. It's odd, because Forte is such a traditional type; if they still had bowler hats, he'd be wearing one—he's a born-again conservative. Yeah", Hamlet added in complacent tones, "I'm more sympathetic to him now. I can see his problems. I bet Mrs F even organized the party for him, to help him break the ice. Yeah, that's how it was, for sure."

I pointed out to Hamlet the resemblance between himself and Forte in his description. Here again we were confronted with the lonely only child in him, "spoilt to death" and unhappy with his parents. There also seemed to be expressed his revulsion at his mother's society parties and her own fashionable but dilettante, and possibly controlling, cultural patronage. A question was forming at the back of my mind about the impact of the family culture on Hamlet—was there really something rotten in the state of Denmark? I asked Hamlet if he thought Forte's problems included his mother and her "powerful personality".

"God, no", he responded in astonishment. "She's not shocked by anything—not like my mother. It could be she's a bit heavy for Forte, of course, a bit too dynamic. No, I had a really serious conversation with her. I've got an idea she wants to write an article about me—she saw my play at Christmas—said she could see straight away I was going places. 'Art must come first', she said, and I said that's just what I said! I told her it was bugging me that my talent might get diluted by hereditary considerations, and how I needed to get the status quo off my back—Funny thing is . . ."

I interrupted this drivel to ask Hamlet to define more precisely the difference between Mrs Forte and his own mother.

"Well, for a start, you can really talk to her", he explained confidentially. "I told her all about my problems with Ophelia and she said she could help—she knows a good clinic, a new one, none of this filthy back-street stuff that's still hanging on, and it would all be over in ten minutes. Oh yeah—and the funny thing was, she knew an amazing amount about psychoanalysis. She was really well informed. I'm sure she must have tried it herself, or some sort of therapy. She knew I was in analysis, of course, and said it was a wonderful opportunity for self-observation. I said yes it was, just way out. 'Sit here', she said, sinking into a pile of cushions with her joint, 'sit here and tell me all about it. First of all, what school are you under?' And you won't believe it, Dr Horacio, but my tongue completely seized up. I was fazed, I felt completely gormless. It's never happened to me before. I thought, she'll think I'm a complete phoney, a freak. I know what you're going to say—what can I expect if I get stoned out of my mind? But she was very understanding—said we'd carry on our talk another time, because she could see I was no tame talent, I was really screwed up and obscure . . ."

I was disturbed at the extent to which Hamlet had evidently felt intimidated by this predatory mother-of-Grendel figure, and at the same time flattered by her seductive attentions. Certainly she seemed to represent a caricature of his mother with her patronage of young artists. I could sense, through Hamlet, how flattering it did indeed appear. What disturbed me, as Hamlet gave his account, was the possibility that this woman could seriously interfere with the analysis. If Hamlet became her protégé, she could choose either to patronize or surreptitiously to attack him or indeed myself through the media—my work, my private life. Such journalistic assaults by professional snoopers were not uncommon in the field. It was well known that those who had "tried" analysis and been unable to discover any capacity for passionate experience became either enemies or apostles of psychoanalysis; and it was hard to tell which was the more damaging.

Hamlet had told Mrs Forte "all about" Ophelia. This was unfortunate. I was relieved, for the time being, when he then described how he had been unable to say a word about me or the analysis. I suggested to Hamlet that his tongue had "seized up" as a means of protecting areas that he wanted to keep private. There was a discrepancy between this and saying he could "really talk" to her.

"It was because I was stoned", he insisted sulkily. "You don't know what that does to you. I mean, it's not my scene at all, I'm not habituated. You're such an old romantic with your fancy theories. Anyway I *could* talk—I told her about Ophelia, didn't I? And she understood perfectly—not like my mother."

Clearly he was not sufficiently aware of the intentions behind Mrs Forte's seductions to be on his guard. My anxiety increased, and I asked him whom he believed to be more sincerely concerned for his and Ophelia's welfare—his mother or this woman. He mumbled crossly that it was a stupid question: Mrs Forte didn't know Ophelia, she wasn't at the party—but that made her advice more genuine and impartial. The whole "set-up" was different. She didn't have "designs" on him like his own family. I pointed out that not only had he suspected her of "designing" the entire party, such that the professionalism of the occasion made him feel he and his friends were being used, rather than entertained, for the satisfaction of Mrs Forte's own "trendy" ambitions; but also, Hamlet had clearly experienced her interrogation as that of a witch-like figure who wanted to squeeze from him his deepest and dirtiest secrets, "screwed up and obscure". Moreover, his tongue seizing up suggested he felt he had in some way betrayed Ophelia to outside interference—that it was in fact none of Mrs Forte's business. His feelings of guilt about Ophelia made him vulnerable to this sort of interference.

"Why shouldn't I get advice from an older woman?" he snapped, increasingly irritated. "It seems to me that was just the right thing to do. And she does at least live in the real world of today. My mother inhabits a different planet."

The "different planet", I said, was the field of intimate relationships. Different values pertained to these, such as existed in his own family or in the Polack family, from those in the world of non-intimate relationships—fashion, status, power, et cetera—as represented here by his picture of Mrs Forte and possibly the whole Forte "set-up" as it had impressed itself on Hamlet.

"At least, in the Forte set-up, I didn't feel like something the dog brought in", he said in self-justificatory growl. "It makes a change to feel *welcome* somewhere."

He had, I suggested, been looking for an alternative analyst to me, a seductive substitute for mental pain. It was here in the consulting-room, in the context of his intimate inner world, that he felt "unwelcome".

"Well, yeah" he flashed, "it's true I was getting sick of being railed at and abused by you the whole time!"

He was the lonely Forte–child, I said, and I was the Mrs Forte witch–mummy who was trying to abuse his talents for my own ends. The fact that Mrs Forte was a woman, who perhaps ought to "welcome" feelings and care about his girlfriend or himself, seemed to have particularly intimidated him. Indeed, he had seemed to find his own attack on "feminine" or intimate values reflected in her, making him prey to her seductions—a species of emotional blackmail. But, as his tongue "seizing up" had showed, he had also, in another part of himself, interpreted her interest as being essentially anti-analytic and had used this means to preserve his intimacy. But he still regarded this episode of word-failure in the light of a humiliation. "What are you, some kind of a sadist?" he scowled. "Or is it just your obsession with digging up material for your scientific papers? It's really you, not Mrs Forte, who can't resist displaying your theories in journalese. Just remember, whatever you write, maybe it's *you* who's inventing the whole thing!"

He slouched off in a prickly, ugly mood, quite different from the dozy benevolence of his arrival. He never did tell the "awful" dream he mentioned at the beginning, and I suspected it only existed in the form of the interrogation by Mrs Forte. As I went next-door to soothe myself with a cigarette, I reflected on my own peculiar agitation during this session. His tongue seizing up had been in a sense a manifestation of his faith in me and the analysis. Yet the more I had insisted on this, the more ground I felt I was losing to the enemy. Was that the problem . . . "the enemy"? Had I attacked Mrs Forte too personally, rather than interpreting her significance in the transference? Certainly I had felt a strong personal antagonism to this woman I didn't even know. Was this because she seemed to represent for me, as for Hamlet, certain aspects of his mother, which I could not bear to believe were really part of her character? I must, I thought, get a better hold of myself and my technique in this sensitive situation.

And, during the next session, I had to struggle hard to submit to my own warning. Hamlet arrived swollen with sanctimonious elation, looking very much "mad, bad, and dangerous to know", and announced that he had had a bitter row with Ophelia over the question of an abortion.

"She's got the same obstinacy as her brother but obviously hasn't got even his wits—and they're spread thin enough on the ground. I explained everything to her—as long as she gets on with it now, it's quick, it's easy, it's painless. The more she arses about pulling silly faces, the worse it's going to be. It's completely crazy. I've found out everything about it—this place where it's all absolutely aboveboard, everything is clean and respectable, no questions asked—in fact, nobody need even know, who doesn't already, that is. *That*, of course, is half our problem: instead of telling me straight in the first place, so we could sort it out honestly together, she's gone blurting it out like a baby to the world and his wife—her old fool of a father, my besotted mother and her doting parasite—the whole lot of them. And Nando, of course—he knows too."

Perhaps, I suggested, Ophelia did not require "explaining to" but questioning about her own feelings. We could see from Hamlet's tyrannical language that he was back in the Mousetrap mentality again. Now, he was behaving as though Ophelia and their parents were ganging up to mousetrap *him*. This was the paranoid consequence of his own attack on his parents in the Mousetrap, which involved holding Ophelia up to ridicule. Now it seemed to him that, through this pregnancy, she was taking revenge on him and on his creative adaptation of Shakespeare.

"Well, it's screwing *her* up as much as me!" he continued, with unabated dogmatism. "The fact is, I need to get this sorted out once and for all so it doesn't keep getting in the way of our relationship. I said to her . . . let's look at this rationally . . . does she really *want* to have the bloody thing? Be tied down for the rest of her life, say goodbye to her musical career—because if she drops out now, she'll never make it, she'll be a leftover. And when I *did* ask her straight out—'do you want to have it?'—she said she 'didn't know'! So there you are—it's not even as though she wanted it, she can see quite well it would be lunatic!"

Hamlet's own manner was triumphantly "lunatic"; even by his standards, he was speaking with extraordinary speed and excitability. I found I was interrupting him as much to slow him down as to get him to listen. What, I asked, was the "it" that was "screwing Ophelia up"—was it the pregnancy, or was it perhaps him? In a manner familiar to us, he had interpreted Ophelia's "don't know" answer in terms of his own assumptions. He was looking for proof that she didn't want it, not for evidence of her feelings; nor had he taken account of his own bullying tone and the distorting effect this might have on her answer.

"I just told her the honest truth! If it doesn't come out now, we'll all pay for it later—can you deny that?"

What was his honest intention, I asked—did he sincerely wish to discover what Ophelia's feelings were, or was his "honesty" really intended to prevent himself from finding out?

"Perhaps you should have *her* in analysis if you're so keen to find out", he hissed sarcastically; "you won't believe what *I* say." Then he continued with a self-righteous air, as if controlling his justifiable rage: "All right, if you really want to know, I'll tell you precisely, in plain terms, how it was. After I'd explained everything, she went very quiet and gave me some peculiar looks. She was obviously considering my argument carefully, because she didn't disagree in any way (and what was there to disagree about?—the facts are plain; it's obvious what has to be done). I told her I wanted her to know that in spite of all this pregnancy thing, I was still really keen on her. The last thing we wanted was to wreck our relationship at this point. And I appreciated she could do with some time on her own, to take it all in, so after that I left her— I didn't want to be insensitive. The thing is, when she quietened down and just sat there looking at me, I realized how fond I was of her, and I told her I just couldn't wait for us to shove this big shadow out the way so we could get back together again. Then she smiled and looked almost like the old Ophelia. I promised I'd see her today so we could fix it up. So . . . in the circumstances", concluded Hamlet with a crazy triumph, ". . . I've done everything I possibly could. Especially when you consider that the brat probably isn't mine anyway—I'm just the one to take responsibility!"

Yes, I thought, focusing on his last remark—that was at the root of his entrenched mania. Confirmation was growing for this predominant anxiety. This was his "big shadow". I asked him for his evidence for suspecting the child was not his.

"Evidence!" he laughed scornfully. "I can tell you she wasn't a virgin when *I* had her—and it was easy enough to get her into bed! Do you want to know the evidence for that too? Or am I supposed to call up witnesses? What can I do to satisfy your scientific Honour?"

I reminded him of the early stages of his relationship with Ophelia—the Batman Dream of sweeping her off her feet, the "fuck, fuck" poem, which was really his own romantic vision of opening her "ventages" to a new and blissful world of erotic experience. Clearly his discovery that she was not a virgin had undermined his romantic role as he had conceived it. His anxiety was that instead of being the first to awaken her desire, she had gone to bed with him easily out of habit, an easy lay—the "secret whore" of his phantasy. Not being a virgin also meant that she was experientially in a position to compare his performance with that of other men. Doubts about his own success as a lover then aroused suspicions that she had continued to have other lovers.

This suggestion, of course, enraged him further. "What's it to me if she did or didn't?" he cried. "It's beneath my dignity to interrogate her—like you would if you had the chance."

I told him he was not prepared to be compared with anyone else; it was an assumption of his princely mentality that with his genius and attributes, he was simply not in the same league as other men—he was incomparable.

"Is it too much to expect straightforward honesty from a woman? Do I have to 'have suspicions' and grub about in the dirt just so I can satisfy you with some cheap romantic slurp?"

His own romantic view of Ophelia's virginity had led him to another type of dishonesty, I said—the dishonesty of not expressing his doubts to Ophelia. Had he considered her position, deprived of any chance to understand his hostility?

"Ophelia, Ophelia!" he interjected scathingly. "You seem mighty concerned about Ophelia. How d'you think *I* feel, with all this hanging over me?"

I said I thought he felt let down by this pregnancy, no longer in control of events and of Ophelia in particular. The directorial "fuck fuck" side of himself had been undermined by something that suddenly brought into focus all his doubts about Ophelia's appreciation of him as a lover and about the quality of her love for him. These were linked in his mind with his doubts about the parentage of the baby. Yet, instead of discussing this with her, he had merely harangued and bullied her, just as he had his mother earlier. In effect, he was demanding that she get rid of the baby to prove she belonged only to him—just as he had demanded that Gertrude must get rid of the usurper Claude.

"So what are you really saying?", he snapped sarcastically, "that she ought to have it after all? And then, I suppose, we'll live Happy Ever After! For God's sake, Dr Horacio—get real! How could a couple at our stage in life make it lumbered with a baby? Isn't it time you stopped tilting at windmills?"

Neither of them, I insisted, had even set out on the road at the end of which a decision might be possible. They had not begun to consider what it "meant" to each of them to have the baby aborted or—as Hamlet put it—to "shove this big shadow out of the way". I reminded him of his recent Mousetrap Dream with its clear expression of taking revenge by killing the baby inside the mother. There was the sincere or truthful meaning of his wanting Ophelia to have the abortion. (It occurred to me here that that dream probably also expressed his own fear that somehow he had caused his mother to have abortions in the past, leaving him an only child, like Forte.)

"Oh, come on", he said contemptuously. "The *reality* of this fucking abortion is that it's not a baby at this stage, just a blob of cells. The important thing is, to do it quickly."

The words of Lady Macbeth, I reminded him. This emphasis on precipitate action—"doing it quickly"—was, as he well knew, aimed at preventing thinking from taking place. He used the word "reality" as if it were the explanation to end all questions. Our concern was to identify the emotional reality, not the biological reality. We already had evidence of his tendency to split Ophelia into outside and inside, upper and lower parts, as his means of convincing himself that he controlled her movements and her meaning. This omnipotent attitude of his had been challenged by the pregnancy, and therefore, I believed, a new and uncontrollable jealousy had been awoken in him.

Hamlet received this renewed interpretation of "jealousy" with snorts of unutterable contempt and left at the end of the session more defiant and sanctimonious than ever. I was the one who would suffer (he implied) from my own perversity in not accepting his honest explanations of the best course of action, and my persistence in an old-fashioned romantic viewpoint.

* * *

He was mildly surprised when (as he reported at the next session) Ophelia told him to "sod off"—their relationship was over, and she would never speak to him again. But it failed utterly to dent his mania. He said it merely confirmed his suspicion that the "real" father was "Forte or somebody" after all, and he'd been a fool to be so willing to assume responsibility. If she wanted to blame the right man, that was OK by him. He'd done his duty.

"She had a nerve taking that self-righteous tone with *me*", he concluded. "It could have been Nando, for all I know—he's been screwing her for years and that's a fact—so why not?"

Probably, I suggested, he was making this assumption as a result of his own earlier homosexual relationship with Nando. Had he asked himself for any actual evidence for this "fact", as he called it?

He gave a coarse, barking laugh and said it was "obvious—what do you think brothers and sisters do together? If I'd had a sister to practise on I'd have done the same."

"Obvious", I repeated—there he went again!

"Yes, obvious, obvious!" he almost shouted. And so it went on. By the end of the session my hand was itching with the impulse to clout him. So when I stood up as he left, after opening the door I kept my arms pinioned firmly to my sides. He noticed this.

"Krup–ke!" he said in a military bark, raising his fingers in an ambiguous salute before slithering round the corner.

I was left troubled, and puzzled, by my inability to make any headway with him, or to bring him in touch with his own emotional state. Again I felt I had somehow lost credibility with him through engaging in partisan debate. Despite support from the evidence of his previous dreams, the transference had again become obscured by what he saw as my moral preaching—my hostility to his tyranny, my urgency that he should repair his relationship with Ophelia. My own desire, as he had seen, was that they should have the baby; did this, perhaps, colour all my interpretations? If so, it might explain why he had seemed impervious to them. I was "Krupke" again, the authoritarian (and rather stupid) moralizer—no longer the analyst.

For two weeks we continued in this situation of deadlock.

Meanwhile I reviewed the last sessions, and the entire Mousetrap episode, in my mind, and bit by bit I structured the situation for him. We went over the attack on his mother in the Mousetrap Dream and his princely attitude to Ophelia in the Batman Dream and how he regarded her as his possession. He had deviously engineered the pregnancy as proof of this, and he was likewise trying to engineer the abortion as a test of her love for him. She must prove her willingness to abandon everything else for his sake. But his plans had backfired: the event of the pregnancy had come instead to seem like Ophelia's revenge on him, having awoken hidden doubts and fears about her love for him and his stature as a lover in her eyes, particularly as she was resisting his demands for an abortion. Hence the ugliness of his behaviour towards her. And, I explained to Hamlet, all this derived from his own infantile competitiveness with his creative internal parents— with aspects of Polack, Claude, Gertrude, Shakespeare—and above all with myself in the transference as his analytic father. This first became evident in the Mousetrap, which was intended to rival the genius of Shakespeare but in fact—as he only realized afterwards—merely held up to ridicule the woman he loved. It resulted directly in the pregnancy, another effort to secure her by a display of all-powerful creativity, which had also failed. The demand for an abortion was his next attempt in the same line.

As the complete pattern of this manic episode of acting-out unfolded itself in all its inevitability, with its increasing focus on the analysis as a creative process envied and attacked by his little-boy rivalry, Hamlet's wild fury and accusations gradually gave way to periods of quiet and gloomy depression. I began to feel that I was slowly but steadily regaining some of the ground lost by my own excitability over the Mousetrap. Then one day Hamlet arrived looking altered, pale and slightly shaken. He had had a dream, which he compared to a childish nightmare, though at the time it had not seemed childish but deadly serious.

In the dream *he was walking along a high coastal path* (such as he knew from childhood holidays in the West Country), *when he suddenly had the intimation that he was being followed by a wild beast, which he knew to be a bear. The terrifying thing was that the bear's long shadow was in advance of it, so that Hamlet found himself walking and then running in the shadow.*

> *"As who, pursued with yell and blow,*
> *Still treads the shadow of his foe."*

He felt impelled to glance backwards to see if the bear was nearly upon him, and at that moment fell into a deep hole like a well, landing flat on his back. He realized then, as he looked upwards, that the well was a newly dug grave;

"and I
Was lying on a bed of bones, my mouth
Bunged chokingly with dirt. In panic I flung
The bones in handfuls upwards, but they showered
Down again and hit me about the head.
In revulsion I wept, and through my tears
Noticed in the corner of the grave
A skull, or so I thought, that took on flesh
And spoke to me through rosy smiling lips,
'Climb on my back, young man, and tears shall be
Your recreation.' I climbed on the back
Of the funny old woman and she set me gently down
On the turf at the grave's brink. But still I wept
Incessantly, in floods, and as the waters
Rose below me, there I saw floating
Ophelia, garlanded with flowers, her clothes
Spread wide in the aqueous element, and drinking
Greedily its moisture. And as she grew
Heavier, she sang a mermaid's song, like one
Natively endowed with that condition."

I was astounded by the unanticipated depth of feeling "welling up" out of this "Grave Dream", which for so many weeks Hamlet had prevented from breaking through. Here was the "big shadow" of the threatened baby (as Hamlet had earlier described it), taking the vengeful bear-shape, which caused Hamlet to "fall" out of his impenetrable omnipotence into a "grave" condition. There was even, in the dream, a clear indication that this could be the site of his repentance and "recreation" through tears.

I was intrigued by the "funny old woman"; Hamlet said she reminded him of those disguised "good fairies" in fairy-tales. I agreed that she seemed to be, as it were, the opposite number to the Mrs Forte–witch who presided over abortions; and that the dream generally showed a greater appreciation of femininity than we had seen before in his dreams. For the first time, we had a clear glimpse of Hamlet's maternal transference to me in the analysis, his baby-like dependence. It was an encouraging development—quite different in quality from his initial automatic dependence on me, which derived from the prince in him lacking a confidante.

* * *

The session after this, however, Hamlet came in with the news that Ophelia had had an abortion. He had spent the previous night at the house that Nando shared with Forte and others in Islington, in order to avoid seeing his parents when he came down from Cambridge for his appointments with me. Nando had told him that Ophelia was "no longer pregnant, so he needn't worry about that any more". To his surprise, this news filled Hamlet with an explosive fury, and he demanded to "thrash" Nando at a game of squash. They went out and played for two hours, during which Hamlet was thoroughly beaten by Nando (by far the better player). He said that the game had greatly relieved him.

Hamlet had not, in fact, seen Ophelia since the crazy interview he had recounted to me. She was not well, he said in low and guilt-ridden tones, and was staying at home. He knew that she truly hated him. He didn't need to ask anyone that, he could sense it; besides she had told him as much. But now he had a new goal in life, which was to beat Nando at squash, and he had arranged to play with him on a regular basis.

CHAPTER SIX

The Winter's Tale

QUEEN: Her clothes spread wide,
And mermaid-like awhile they bore her up,
Which time she chanted snatches of old lauds,
As one incapable of her own distress,
Or like a creature native and indued
Unto that element.

[IV. vii. 174–179]

By the time he learned of Ophelia's abortion and illness, Hamlet's demeanour had already commenced its sea-change from the Mousetrap mania. He became subdued and depressed, and this depression, in the context of the analytic work, had produced the fascinating Grave Dream. After this, he was often silent for long periods during sessions, and for many weeks oscillated between withdrawal, depression, and paranoia. He made decided efforts to cooperate in the analysis, coming on time to the sessions and bringing whatever he could remember in the way of dreams. These were invariably repetitive "grave dreams" on the lines of his being imprisoned in the dark some-where, with only small windows for eyes on the world, despairing of release. None of them had the emotional depth of the original Grave Dream. There was, however, a new element, which linked back to that dream and his falling into the grave—it was his strong identification with the aborted baby. He experienced him-self as having similarly been flung into the rectum, discarded, to await evacuation.

Hamlet was not under the tutorship of Professor Polack dur-ing this term. I gathered he was doing very little work, and he seemed to have given up most of his extra-curricular activities, apart from a fanatical adherence to playing squash with Nando whenever he was in London. This was the only area in which he manifested any spark of vitality. It meant that when he came to his sessions, he had usually either played or was about to play squash. It was his ambition, he said, to become good enough to beat Nando at the game.

"Nando belongs to a private sports club with fabulous facili-ties. And actually he's a bloody good teacher in his way. One of these days I shall really beat the hell out of him. That's why I've taken up meat-eating again. I need to build myself up. Anyway, everybody's going vegetarian these days, it's just a fad with them, not a principle."

He saw fighting Nando as a means of both punishing and rebuilding himself. Frequently, over the next month or two, I tried to explain to him that it was also a way of avoiding confronting his feelings. He was out of touch with his vengeful jealousy of Nando (who represented Ophelia's lover in his eyes), which was his real motive for fighting him. Above all, he was out of touch with his anxiety that he had intruded on Ophelia, killing her baby.

The news about Ophelia was not good. She had officially taken leave of absence from her studies, because she was suffering from severe depression and had twice tried to slit her wrists. Afraid of leaving her alone at all, her father had arranged for her to spend a period in hospital, where she was in a ward amongst (mainly) anorexic girls.

"Nando says being in with that lot would drive anyone off their rocker even if they weren't crazy before", said Hamlet grimly. "He says the only advantage is, she can't slit her wrists.

He makes it sound like some kind of a joke, but underneath I know he thinks I'm a real shit." He spoke in a flat, dull tone, as though he were religiously making himself report the entire un-savoury truth—and he proceeded, putting his sentences together with an effort:

"I can never face Polly again either. It's his own stupid fault. Why did he have to get so idiotically excited over any old trashy thing I'd written? He was even disappointed when I gave up writing for that obsolete rag *Varsity*. He expected me to leap through the hoops like a performing monkey to boost his own fading ego. Same as Claude—just to make me feel guilty. Why should I be his instrument, or anybody's? And now they've landed me in this mess."

Hamlet's tone was one of gloomy complaint. Clearly he was somehow blaming Professor Polack's attitude to his work for stimulating a false excitement, a showing-off, in his own relation to Ophelia. I did wonder if he had felt he was unable to live up to Polack's expectations (which seemed to have been a little ideal-ized), rather as he had turned against his father, though it looked as though this idealization had bored rather than daunted him. In some way it had damped his interest, in the tutor and possibly in the subject. Hamlet agreed with this:

"It was his fault for making me into something I wasn't. It just showed how out of touch he was, like Claude—a complete dino-saur. As if I was something out of Pseuds Corner."

Now that the pressure of his claustrophobic identification with his "uncle–father" had been relieved, I said, he was plunged into a persecutory depression. He felt a "pseud", a dinosaur, ridicu-lous—stimulated and encouraged by these fathers, only to be laughed at afterwards for being merely a little boy. His own sexual activity seemed unrelated to the possibility of his ever join-ing the ranks of true fatherhood.

"What you mean is", he said moodily, "I'm a lousy, degen-erate, inconsiderate slob. You can say it. Can I help it if that is my nature?"

Here, as repeatedly during this period, he sought reassurance from me that I, at least, could see his better nature—that he was only the victim of himself. But his self-blame and self-denigration, I explained, was not the same thing as taking responsibility for his own feelings and actions. This was where our problem lay—in convincing him of the value of feelings, his own and other people's.

"What is it you want me to do, then?" he countered in a more irritable tone. "Grovel in front of them all—shave my head and put on a hair shirt, sleep on a bed of nails? Next you'll be saying I'm disappointing *your* expectations, like the rest of them. Well, perhaps my talents just aren't up to it after all."

Again, I repeated gently, it was not a case of doing but of feeling. I suggested that the "expectations" he was afraid he could never fulfil were not those of "winning" (action), as when he played squash with Nando, but of emotional communication. He seemed aware that in this area he had a lack of talent. And we could see that his sense of disappointing his father and Polack was now devolving upon me—that I was the one he felt he'd really disappointed.

"Well, wasn't it you who was egging me on over the whole business with Ophelia?" he turned on me accusingly, at last. "You can't deny, you were keen to have us married off as soon as possible—is it any wonder I took the shortest road? And you could see all along I was going to make a fool of myself over the play, but you never did anything to stop me, did you?"

I said he felt I had not been firm enough to protect him, to contain his little-boy destructive mania. Owing to my weakness, he felt, he had become vulnerable to destructive aspects of himself. The play, the baby, the abortion—now plunged him into the depths of worthlessness; he had crashed. This had been anticipated up to a point in the "To be or not to be" Dream. It was not an accident, but the inevitable conclusion to acting-out. Yet it still seemed to be his sense of humiliation—"making a fool of himself"—that was paramount. And now he was searching for solutions in the form of action—looking for something to "do"—to set this right.

"But as far as the baby goes, I'm still not sure it *was* me—even now", he complained.

I reminded him of how the emotional reality was a separate issue from the genetic paternity, as we'd discussed before. It was what he felt he had done to Ophelia and others in his mind that meant he couldn't face them.

"You mean, I'm to blame, whether it was me or not", he said quickly, with a hint of paranoia.

No, I said, I meant that his feelings of guilt were proportional to the damage that he *really felt* he had caused. And I reviewed with him once again how he felt his sexual relations with Ophelia had begun badly, intrusively, as in the Batman Dream and his "fuck fuck" poem; how she had perhaps not felt his "governing her ventages" to be the blissful experience he had expected; how her pregnancy had therefore seemed to be none of his doing; and how her abortion had confirmed his suspicion of his own worthlessness. Hence in the Grave Dream, the bear–baby had turned in revenge and chased him into the grave of deep depression, where he was now. This was the emotional reality in his mind, and this was what he had difficulty in facing.

"So what am I supposed to do?", he said with a tinge of repulsion. "Say I didn't mean it, shall we have another go?—with my unsuitable genes? I mean, if it *was* mine, she obviously thought it wasn't worth having, didn't she."

I told him he was feeling identified with the baby—thrown out for being worthless. He had wanted Ophelia first to get pregnant, then to have the abortion, to prove she belonged to him. But, instead, he felt he had become the victim of her revenge—that she had turned and aborted *him*. It was not "unsuitable genes" that troubled him, but the painful feeling that he was an intruder who had been discovered masquerading as a provider of babies and been thrown out.

He was silent for a few minutes, then resumed his complaint in pained tones: "What I can't understand", he said, "was how she did it—arranged it, I mean. I can't believe Polly had anything to do with it. That means it must have been Nando, the supercilious slob—or Nando and Forte between them. Which is proof that it wasn't my child." He added, with a revived bitterness, "I expect he's laughing at me even now. But I've been practising at Cambridge too, and when I see him tonight I'll really murder him!"

It was hard, indeed, to convince Hamlet that ultimately there was no substitute for the reality of feeling. A very delicate balance existed throughout this period between his gradual, tentative approach to painful feelings in the analysis and his belief that action would do instead of confronting the feelings—as in the squash-playing. I reminded him of how he had said that Nando had used his sister for "practising" sex; now he was "practising" squash, as if this could provide the solution to a painful and confusing emotional problem.

Then, in a new tone of genuine perplexity, he said: "Did she agree to do it to spite me—to show me how worthless I am? Or did she let herself be bullied by those buggers? I just can't understand her!"

I said his "not understanding", which he had now repeated twice, was an achievement in itself. Before, he had just regarded Ophelia as an instrument in his own show; now he spoke as though her motives were not as obvious as her attributes. Perhaps, like the "baby", which had also been unreal to him, she had something inside her that he accepted was not known by him—her own heart of mystery.

"But you see", he explained, "I *did* know about her, that was the whole point—I knew her from a little girl, and her family, her music, and everything. I knew exactly who she was from the beginning."

But this "knowing about", I said, was, of course, quite different from "knowing" her intimately in depth—her feelings, motives, desires. We had discussed before his frustration at discovering that sexual relations did not somehow explain everything after all.

He paused for a few moments, ruminating; then he began to recount what he had never told me before—his first proper meeting with Ophelia. "The funny thing was", he began, "she was around all the first year, of course, and I knew who she was, but I never really *noticed* her. Even at Polly's, she was always hidden away in a corner, mouse-like, usually with a friend or something—you never saw her on her own. Then one evening I bumped into her coming out of the laundrette at the bottom of the hill near Kettle's Yard. She had a plastic bag of laundry in each hand; she reminded me of those French paintings of milkmaids. I had a pile of dirty jumpers in my arms because I'd been told this place still had a dry-cleaning machine. I'd never been there before. She recognized me as she came out and said, 'You should wash those by hand, Hamlet', and gave me a very strange, mysterious smile, slightly mocking. It was the first time she'd called me by my name, all the time I'd been in Cambridge. Then she put a bag on each handlebar and wobbled off up the hill back to college. I watched her till she got to the top, all the time thinking to myself, What did she mean? What did she really mean?"

I was interested to hear this description of a more enigmatic, Mona-Lisa-like Ophelia in Hamlet's eyes, who had surprised him by not appearing "mouse-like" and who aroused his curiosity rather than his omnipotence. There was also a hint of his often-denied romanticism in the "milkmaid" image. It was a view of Ophelia that seemed to have been buried by the Mousetrap affair, or possibly one that had only occurred to Hamlet in retrospect, in the sense of imaginative memory rather than mechanical recall. The self-questioning was definitely a hopeful sign, possibly a way out of his present impasse. I began to feel we were back on firm analytic ground. Perhaps, I suggested to him, we could see here a first step towards his questioning his own sincerity and examining where his own personal worth really lay, rather than pessimistically condemning himself as "worthless", as though this were an inevitable feature of his genetic makeup.

But he responded gloomily that all this was a "pointless exercise. You can't bring back love—that's gone. All that's left is a sort of detached feeling, scientific. Diagnosing the cause of death."

* * *

And so it went on in the analysis for many weeks, with Hamlet showing no interest in making any inquiries about why Ophelia had had the abortion, and correspondingly maintaining his own static position in the "grave" of dead relationships, where nothing was expected from him in terms of communication. It was hard work trying to awaken his capacity to look back and question his own motives and sincerity in the past—all was "pointless" and "hopeless". He preferred to wrap himself in pessimism. The Grave was the only secure and comfortable situation to be in, and of course he was reluctant to be disturbed. At the same time I was impressed by his new dependence on me and by the development of the transference. Elements of both his father and Polack were now regularly gathered into me, and his struggle with them— especially his sense that he had disappointed them—became focussed more inside the analysis. But even more important was the maternal transference, which had first shown itself in the Grave Dream. This was now becoming more firmly established, in relation to the baby who thinks he's been weaned because he bit the nipple. This fierce, domineering baby-within-Hamlet took us back also to the Ghost Dream and the source of male aggression against his mother that was expressed in it. Then, in the last session, he had accused me (perhaps with some justification? I wondered) of not being strong enough to contain his aggression during the Mousetrap. The extent to which this was directed against me as his analytic mother was now becoming much clearer. He truly felt that I carried the scar of his aggression.

Then one evening Hamlet came in flushed and excited, announcing in the same breath that he had beaten Nando in a game of squash and had had a dream.

In this dream, *he was in a submarine with his friends from the play—Rosenfeld, Gildstein, Seaman, and Peacock. They were taking the submarine "on a trip to Hertford to be reconditioned". It seemed quite natural that the way to Hertford was under water. But then they started fighting over who was in control of the vessel, and Hamlet was afraid it was going to crash. He realized it was vitally important to save the "black box" and take it to Hertford so they could see what was going wrong with the submarine. But he could not get the importance of this over to his friends, who continued "arsing about", so he seized the black box and escaped from the upper hatch.*

It was not quite clear in the dream whether the danger was caused by the friends fighting for control or whether there was something inherently wrong with the vessel. Hamlet saw easily enough that the dream described his own need to be "reconditioned" after the fiasco of the Mousetrap, with the friends representing his own masturbatory fingers generating delusions of omnipotence. And the "crash" described his own sudden deflation (with possibly some reference to drugs and Forte's party, and "tripping"). But he seemed to recognize the need to get help from "Hertford" and to provide the information about his inmost functioning, which was contained in the black box.

Clearly, there was a pun in the name "Hertford" on the lines of something like "heartfelt", which could be linked to our discussions about sincerity. Hamlet's dream diagnosed his illness in terms of the need to get out of an enclosed state, back to a condition of real emotionality at the "heart of his mystery" (the black box)—not a status-conscious identity such as that stimulated by the "Mrs Forte" model of achievement with its "tripping" and "crashing", "arsing about" irresponsibly. In the dream he had had to make a choice between opposing sets of values. Also, as in the original Grave Dream, these values indicated that he could not do it all by himself, in his usual directorial manner. Yes, I thought, this Submarine Dream confirmed that the analysis was under way again.

Hamlet then said that he had another association to the dream. There was a nurse on Ophelia's ward named Sister Hertford, whom Nando had mentioned. In fact, said Hamlet, Ophelia was said to be much better and was due to come out of hospital next week. He said this almost reluctantly, with some apprehension, and when I pointed this out to him, he confessed that he was terrified of accidentally encountering her. There was "no question" of a deliberate meeting, of course. He had felt a gloomy satisfaction at the thought that she was restrained in the ward under supervision, while he was at the same time paying his regular penitential visits to me in my secluded basement. He would have preferred this arrangement to go on indefinitely, for ever.

Now she would be loose in the world again, and even though he knew they would try to avoid each other, his security was gone and his passive morbid resignation might no longer rest unchallenged. He couldn't quite see why, since he had neither hope nor desire of ever resuming their relationship. Yet his dream had suggested that he had in mind some presiding "nursing" or healing figure who was common to both of them and who could read the "black boxes" of both him and Ophelia—perhaps on the lines of this Sister Hertford or of the old woman in the Grave Dream who had said, "tears shall be your recreation".

* * *

In the session after this, Hamlet told me that his mother had been to visit Ophelia. In fact, she had been several times, but he had never spoken directly to her about it. But Nando told him casually that Gertrude had left a bowl of daffodil bulbs for Ophelia to take with her when she came out, and Hamlet had had a dream about it.

In the dream, *he was walking along what seemed like an interminable labyrinth of dark corridors, behind a woman wearing long white robes and a headdress, perhaps like a nun. Eventually they came to a door, and as the woman stopped to open it, Hamlet saw that she was carrying a bowl of daffodil bulbs newly in flower. The woman entered and shut the door, apparently oblivious to Hamlet's presence. It seemed that he was unable to open the door for himself and was about to turn away in despair when he realized that there was a clear window in the door, so he could at least see inside. When he looked through, he had to blink because the light was dazzling by contrast with the dark corridor. It was a large room with many beds, and he realized this must be the hospital ward where Ophelia was; but the room seemed decorated as if for a party, with bouquets of flowers and ribbons festooned all over it. There was a loud buzz of gay chatter, but when the white-robed woman entered, there was a hush. She put the bowl down on a lace-covered table. Ophelia was standing behind it.*

Then the woman said, "What was lost has now been found", and Ophelia said, gravely, "Welcome, as spring to the earth". And all the girls in the room, in their nightdresses, brought garlands of flowers and hung them on Ophelia. Ophelia jumped up on the bed behind her, holding out her arms, and began to sing:

> *O Proserpina! tell me now*
> > *It is gone, it is gone*
> *How should I a true love know*
> > *From another one?*

> *My spirits followed you down below;*
> > *I was numb, I was numb.*
> *My own soul was the embryo*
> > *And so, undone.*

> *Imprisoned by the winter's flaw*
> > *In the grave, in the grave*
> *Till you unlatched the chamber door*
> > *And my sins forgave.*

> *I never knew how still it was*
> > *In the ground, in the ground*
> *I was nerveless, listless, voiceless,*
> > *Without a sound.*

> *Bound I was by that deadly spell*
>   *Like a stone, like a stone;*
> *You promised me that out of hell*
>   *At last I'd come.*

> *Released by hope I saw that I could*
>   *Let it be, let it be;*
> *Because I would at last reward*
>   *Your faith in me.*

When Ophelia had finished her song, she beckoned two other girls up onto the bed and placed garlands on them, then tossed flowers to others, and they all started to leap from bed to bed exuberantly, giggling and laughing. Meanwhile Hamlet remained with his face rivetted to the window, feeling as though he were "in a courtroom waiting for sentence to be pronounced". He wanted to sneak away, but his legs would not move. Then to his horror the woman with the daffodils started to walk towards him, and he turned and ran back away down the corridor.

This, then, was the beginning rather than the end of Hamlet's "recreation". After he had recounted the dream, he was quiet and thoughtful. I asked him why he had been "horrified" when the woman walked towards him—was he expecting punishment, or a reprimand from her? He said no, he was terrified that she was coming to let him in, as if she, too, had expectations of him. I suggested these expectations might constitute shame or remorse on his part, and a re-awakening such as he imagined Ophelia to have undergone in his dream. This mental activity was, if sincere, more painful than the self-inflicted carceration of blame or punishment.

Then Hamlet said, stirring awkwardly on the couch, "It's weird, but I feel as if a great weight was pressing down on me. I can't get rid of the feeling left by that dream, it hangs on. In fact, I feel incredibly sleepy. If I stay here, I don't think I can stop myself going to sleep."

He roused himself, however, as it was in fact nearly the end of the session. But before getting up, looking out of the window, he remarked in a tone of wonder "how blue the sky was today". I pointed out, with a heightened interest, that the sky visible from the consulting-room window was in fact grey and heavy. His

vision was a subjective or "dream" one, associated with his looking through the window of the ward at the brightness of the revived condition attained by Ophelia. But whereas in the actual
dream he had felt excluded and disgraced, the bright window in
the consulting-room seemed to offer a prospect on his own regen-
eration. His subjective vision, I felt sure, indicated his hope that
the baby in him could, through the analysis, be rescued from the
grave–rectum. The light might shine on him too and wake him out
of his deep sleep. On this note of resurgent optimism (which later,
alas, I came to view with some modification) we parted, I believed, on the verge of a breakthrough.

The Tempest

HAMLET: Here hung those lips that I have kissed I know not how oft. Where be your gibes now, your gambols, your songs, your flashes of merriment, that were wont to set the table on a roar? Not one now to mock your own grinning? Quite chop-fallen? Now get you to my lady's chamber and tell her, let her paint an inch thick, to this favour she must come.

[V. i. 182–188]

Ophelia came home shortly before the Easter break. I did not see Hamlet for three weeks. On the first session of the new term he came in muffled to the hilt in a long black scarf wound round his neck and ears, dark glasses, and a zipped-up leather jacket. He moved with uncharacteristic slowness and lay down silently and lugubriously. Then from the depths of the scarf came a low, strangled humming. For a moment I wondered whether he was sobbing, but he then explained that he "had a stinking cold and was drowning in catarrh; his brain was buzzing". There was still a question in my mind about the humming, which sounded somehow familiar. I asked him what it was. He didn't seem to realize at first that he had been humming anything specifically and moved his jaws to discover what it was, then said in a tone of mild boredom: "It's just some old Beatles song." I asked which one, and he replied reluctantly, "It's one called 'Help'." When I asked for the words, he said he couldn't remember, so I reminded him they went something like:

> How can you laugh when you know I'm down . . .
> Help! You know I need somebody,
> Help! You know I need someone.

He seemed mildly amused and said, rather contemptuously, "I didn't think you were supposed to divulge your cultural interests." I suggested to him that he was "drowning in catarrh"—namely some flood of emotionality—and had made the significant step of asking me for help, although I had had to fish for the confession.

"Oh, yes—Dr Horacio, fisher of men!" he teased, and broke into a violent fit of coughing, during which he took off his glasses and blew his nose. When I asked why he was wearing the glasses, he said he had a stye in his eye and then, after further prompting, confessed he "couldn't stand people looking straight at him"—he felt intolerably exposed. In fact, he had distanced himself from his group of friends and spent the vacation shut up at home.

"Even old Claude was making an effort—though it was transparent he was acting on instructions from my mother. She'd obviously told him I was 'depressed', so he'd been racking his brains to see what he could do to draw me out of myself, and he came up with the idea of taking me sailing on the Welsh Harp—as if I was a ten-year-old or something. He's just not switched on. But my mother was dead keen for me to go, she practically begged me, so I thought what the hell, it's no big deal anyway, so I went—it was easier than not going. The next day, of course, we both went down with flu." He coughed again and laughed ironically, "Yes, at last we found something in common!"

Nevertheless I pointed this out as perhaps a new turn in their relationship and suggested that Hamlet in some part of himself had appreciated his sympathetic intentions.

"His intentions—O God, his *intentions*! There's always something behind Claude's gestures, he can't do anything
spontaneously. So what, who cares . . . if it suits him to play
Daddy, that's OK by me—even if he hasn't the foggiest idea how
to go about it. At least it keeps my mother quiet."

I also noted that Hamlet's mention of the sailing episode, together with his own appearance, defensively wrapped in leather
and glasses, was reminiscent yet again of the Ghost–pilot. In the
original dream he had found this uniform rather threatening, and
the other time he had imitated it in order to appear threatening
himself; but this time it seemed more of a refuge. He agreed that
what he needed was a refuge; he couldn't face any of the "old
crowd":

"Even people I don't know, I feel, must be staring at me. I
went into Hall on Wednesday for dinner—I hadn't been for
ages—and I could see people—well, *looking* at me, laughing—not
out loud, of course, but I knew what they were thinking."

What did he believe they were thinking?

"Well, I knew they must have been to see that fucking play.
They know all about me, and Ophelia, and everything. They know
exactly what was going on, and they're thinking what a pansy-
faced prick I was to play the whole thing in public, expecting to
get idolized like some tit of a pop star. Why couldn't I keep my
sordid little secrets to myself, like everybody else, then I wouldn't
look such a fool."

He spoke vehemently and contemptuously of himself, ending
with another episode of coughing and sneezing. Then, in a flatter,
more detached tone of voice, he explained that after the sailing
afternoon he had taken to his bed in his new room in his parents'
flat and been content to lie there day after day in a fluey or ex-
hausted state, staring out of the newly installed skylight and
listening to music through headphones plugged firmly over his
ears.

"Fabulous things, clouds", he began, in a theatrical manner,
slightly sarcastic: "the way their shape is always changing. The
frieze of life. You can see them as different characters, or else as the
same character going through a whole succession of experiences.
You know—life events. The really fascinating thing is the total
meaninglessness of it all—the clouds never let you forget that."

The "meaninglessness", I stressed, was an important recognition. He sounded offended at my taking him at his word, saying: "Actually I got down some pretty good poems about it—don't worry, I'm not going to read them to you, I know they're not your style. My mother, of course, would be dying to have a look. She put her head round the door—pretending to see if I wanted dinner or something—saw I was writing—'Oh, Hamlet!' she twitters, 'you're writing again! I'm so glad.' What the hell is she glad for? Good job she can't see what I *do* write. I make quite sure of that."

This was said with a hard determination, making sure I took note. I asked him what he thought would disturb his mother in his poems, and he said she'd "probably think I was going to commit suicide or something—she's so literal-minded. I have to protect her from myself. Anyway, I hope by now she's learned I've got to have my privacy."

I told Hamlet I accepted his despair had to be taken seriously; his sincerity in this was not in doubt. During the holiday when I had not been available he had at least managed to accept the refuge of his parents' home, where he felt he could hide away his intolerable sense of "meaninglessness" and not be assaulted by "humiliation" (as with his fellow-students).

"Well, actually", he said, "it was a relief to get back into digs— I would definitely have died of claustrophobia if I'd lived at home another ten minutes. It was the dreadful way she kept fluttering her eyelashes at me, anxiously, all the time trying not to interfere, not to 'say anything'. And Claude wasn't much better, he's gone kind of soft. 'Untimely death of student—suffocated by pity'."

I hoped, however, that once the analysis was re-established after the usual distancing of the break, we would get more information about the nature of his depression. But it took a surprisingly long time to regain his confidence. Guilt and shame were not enough to explain the restless and persecutory quality of his depression; they did not account for its deep humiliation. Like a suppurating sore, it was aggravated by every slight contact from his intimate friends—in particular every expression of concern. As in the Mousetrap Dream, he felt surrounded by faces "leering and laughing" at him. Consequently he avoided contact with his former circle, shutting himself away in his room or in a remote corner of the library, pretending to work. As if in response to this, he received a note from Professor Polack, inviting him to contribute to a journal whose editorial board he was on.

"Even he feels sorry for me", said Hamlet bitterly. "As always, he's got it all wrong. He thinks I'm burying myself in intellectual pursuits to work off my Great Guilt. The reality is much more crude and basic. I just want to be left alone. I don't want anything to do with any of them. I can't stand their fucking pity. Let them indulge themselves, feeling all warm and compassionate about everybody—it's fine, if that's what turns them on—but leave me out of it. I'm not going to play that game."

He continued in this gloomy and irritable vein for several weeks. His cold, with complications of cough and sinusitis, took a long time to subside, and instead, a virulent rash of spots erupted over his face, beyond anything he had ever suffered before. He remained wrapped in the black scarf as spring progressed. Meanwhile he claimed to be doing no academic work apart from the minimum hack-work with which he could get by without drawing attention to himself. I gathered that he was also writing a great deal of poetry, which, of course, he showed no one, and which he kept in a locked black box—"yeah, like the Submarine Dream", he pre-empted my saying.

And the day after this, he did finally bring a dream that clarified what I felt to be the "suppurating sore" within him:

"I was in this boat with Ros and Gil. Actually it was an Enterprise dinghy like the one I went out in with Claude in the Easter holiday. The idea was that we were going fishing; we had a trawling net over the side. But Ros and Gil were arsing about, moving piles of books from one side of the dinghy to the other, saying they had to get the ballast right, and taking swigs from a bottle of whisky which they kept passing between them. And Ophelia was there too, sitting in the prow of the boat with her sheet of yellow hair spreading out in the breeze. She seemed to be waving and egging them on."

And what was Hamlet himself doing?

"I was at the tiller, so I couldn't move. Then Gil noticed that there was a catch in the net, so I turned the boat into the wind, and we all started to haul with all our strength. In fact, the boat nearly capsized as we got it on board. Ros said, 'Bugger this rotten leaking carcass of a butt'."

Here Hamlet paused uncomfortably, then continued:

"And it turned out to be a man, a black man—I know what you're going to say. But the thing was—not only was he dripping wet, he was covered in seaweed and barnacles. He looked like some weird sea-creature from the depths. Ros and Gil started to pull the net off him, pissing about and making jokes about how he looked 'half fish, half monster'. But now the wind had really got up, and although I had the tiller again it didn't seem to control the boat any more—the sheets were all entangled with the ropes of the net, and the sails were flapping like mad."

And Ophelia?

"Ophelia seemed to have vanished—I never noticed her after the beginning. There was just the mainsail flapping furiously over us, making a terrible din:

> *"The pinioned sail roared loudly overhead,*
> *And foolishly the fishes beat the floor*
> *For kissing of their fins, yet still the ship*
> *Bent on towards its goal. Like unback'd colts*
> *They prick'd their ears, advanced their eyes,*
> *And lifted up their noses, smelling music.*
> *Plunging and tacking through water and air, the boat*
> *Drew them half wading, half flying to the water's edge*
> *Where finally it lodged amongst the reeds."*

This dream, I thought, was a fascinating history or review of Hamlet's sexual awakening: from masturbatory experimentation (his "fingers" represented by Ros and Gil), through discovery of the "monstrous" genitals (like his "black box"), and the sense of being out of control with the "flapping mainsail" taking over the boat/body—Ophelia having turned into the sail and taken on a somewhat frightening aspect. Also, of course, the whole "enterprise" (as in the name of the dinghy class) came under the auspices of the father who had introduced him to it, which made a link with his earlier dreams of the Ghost–pilot and the "hovering" father in the Mousetrap Dream who had tried to discipline his son's mania.

"It was you I called a fisher of men", said Hamlet, coughing. "This is what your fishing trips lead to."

It was more, I said, Hamlet fishing in his own unconscious, to discover lost or unknown parts of himself. As so often before, I reminded him that it was *his* dream—no invention of mine. In this dream he did seem to be revising and repairing his attack on *A Midsummer Night's Dream*; it showed how he had worked his way out of his claustrophobia, carrying further his escape in the Submarine Dream, and becoming this strange barnacled black man. It was clear that this man, like a merman in a fairy tale, was an alter-ego of his own.

"Not simple racism?" he said bluntly.

Possibly racist, I said, but not "simply", any more than the sail was "simply" feminist. Both seemed to represent essential aspects or qualities within himself, vital to the functioning of his "boat": one making a link with undersea richness, the other catching the winds of spiritual movement. As an image of womanhood, I was interested in the persecutory quality of the sail. The expanse of light-catching material (like Ophelia's yellow hair) was reminiscent also of Sister Hertford's flowing white robes in his dream.

"And of my mother in the Mousetrap Dream", he added. "And of Claude, too, if you like, in his fancy silk dressing gown."

In that dream, of course, Gertrude had seemed to collapse under his onslaught, and Claude had given him a stern warning. Whereas here, it was the Ophelia-sail itself that took on the role of somehow rebuking or frightening him. Yet the sail had not actually capsized the boat, nor had the confusion in the boat resulted in Hamlet's having to escape from a hatch, as in the Submarine Dream. In fact, Hamlet pointed out, the boat seemed to have a mind of its own, independent of its human sailors, and they felt themselves irresistibly drawn to the water's edge, which was the boat's goal. Yes, I agreed, it was a dream of discovery rather than of omnipotence: of following desires rather than manipulating excitement. The dream also gave us a clue as to his feeling of rejection by Ophelia for being an ugly barnacle-man: when his identity was finally fished up and exposed to view, he was (he felt) clearly no match for her shimmering sail-beauty.

This was certainly a new and hopeful departure. After Hamlet had left, I had a few minutes' break and walked up to the High Street with the excuse of buying a packet of cigarettes, but really to enjoy the bright spring sunshine. On the way there I indulged myself in feeling pleased, even elated. The tide was turning. On the way back, however, I noticed a certain frustration in myself. I was eager to facilitate Hamlet's recovery, but despite his plea for "help" and his calling me a "fisher of men", I suspected I was a little unnecessary. There was something tenuous about our relationship. We were not working *together*; his dreams were doing all the work, and I did nothing but confirm their significance. If only I could do more to pull him forwards, now that we were on the right track! I felt almost impatient in my optimism.

Then, to the next session, Hamlet brought a dream that seemed to follow on directly from this "Tempest" Dream, filling out its implications regarding his own identity:

"I was lying on the shore, alone. I could feel the mud in my toes and fingers, stretched out. I felt I was pinioned there. I was looking up at the sun filtering through the canopy of leaves overhead, and there was a strange music enveloping me on all sides. I couldn't tell where it was coming from; it seemed to come out of the ground and the air at the same time."

Here again was the idea of music holding the elements of the dream together, providing its meaningfulness. I asked whether the experience seemed pleasurable, or painful.

"Neither", he said emphatically. *"It was paralysing. My senses were all bound up. I couldn't move away, or stop listening. I realized it was a dream. The weird thing was, when I woke up, I remembered the music very vividly, not as a tune but as a physical sensation, and I had this intense longing to get back into the dream. At the same time I knew I was still asleep, but not in that dream. I was still stuck in the mud, and my body was covered in barnacles and seaweed, as though I was growing or rather rotting into the beach like some old piece of driftwood. It was then I realized that I stank. And a voice began to sing my song for me, to the words in my head:*

> *Full fathom five my father lies,*
> *Developing pearl and weed;*
> *Whilst Ros and Gil are under hatches*
> *Safely stoned in bed.*
>
> *The reasonable shore is mud*
> *And I alone am conscious*
> *Now the ooze has belched me up*
> *How infinite my loss.*

In dismay I mourned the change
    I cried to dream again
Without the music sweet and strange
    I'm but a sot like him.

He used to stroke me, taught me how
    To know my words, at first;
My lasting profit is that now
    I know how to curse.

So fill my skin with pinches black,
    Make me strange stuff—
A canker'd, fuming maniac
    A true moon-calf.

The devils hiss me into madness,
    The music must be free;
O Prospero! this thing of darkness
    I acknowledge me.

This heartfelt lament, founded on his identification with the sea-
"monster"–man of the previous dream, filled me with hope about
the possibility of Hamlet's really coming to terms with his own
"darkness" (omnipotence). His realization that he "stank" was an
extension of his barnacle-man identification, and he clearly felt
himself rejected by both Ophelia and the "Prospero" figure, who,
with his emphasis on words, taught him to "curse". In this
Prospero we could see aspects of Polack and of myself in the
analysis, both representing Ophelia's guardian—the father behind
her—who seemed to Hamlet to have pronounced him inadequate.
There was also, of course, a link with his own father, who had
introduced him to the "enterprise". Now, taking the two dreams
together, this masculine element seemed to be more an integral
part of Ophelia herself. This went along with his growing appreciation of the power of femininity. This was the music that "must
be free" (as in the Museum Dream)—a reversal of his old directorial mode. My enthusiasm increased as I felt we were getting
nearer the source of his intense sense of humiliation: was it, then,
Ophelia whom he believed to be always "laughing at him"?

    "Of course, Ophelia is an amazing musician herself", Hamlet
mumbled, clearly finding this latter interpretation extremely un-

comfortable. However, he noted other links with the Winter's Tale Dream, such as Ophelia's hymn to Proserpina as the agent of release from inner darkness, linked with the figure of Sister Hertford (heartfelt). I agreed that he seemed to be making a similar appeal here to myself in the form of "Prospero".

I also showed how the "darkness" or "madness" acknowledged in the dream had expressed itself somatically in the spots on his face, his cold, and his wrapping himself up in the scarf not so unlike a man caught in a net or a piece of driftwood wrapped in seaweed. He squirmed at this, but over the next week or two his health made a noticeable improvement, and he was more cheerful than I had known him. Bedded down in the mud, perhaps he was metabolizing a sea-change. For the Tempest Dream was, I believed, a dream about the making of poetry as well as love, and I wondered whether Hamlet had perhaps been working seriously at his own writing. Certainly I was very hopeful about these signs of a new dependence on creative internal objects who could bring the "music" into his life to transform his own "curses". This would be a genuine mental prosperity.

* * *

However, this was not to be. Our progress was abruptly cut short. Perhaps not so abruptly, for during the final weeks of his analysis I could sense him tiptoeing away, out of contact with me, distancing himself. His manner was pleasant and polite, but he was cocooned in a type of indolence or passivity. The intimacy of the transference, which had been growing so strongly, seemed to evaporate. Indeed, looking back on it, even by the Tempest Dream the transference had lost the maternal quality that had been its most hopeful recent development. Instead of the baby-Hamlet's attachment to his analytic mother, we were back to the little boy wrestling with his analytic father—and now accepting (unwillingly) the impotence of his immaturity. In itself this was, of course, a useful beginning. But this kind of dependence seemed to stimulate an underlying irritation with me, amounting almost to persecution, though not of the old explosive paranoid type, and carefully veiled by politeness. The precise cause puzzled me greatly—was it really that he couldn't stand the painfulness of these new feelings of ugliness and humiliation? He must know— we all did—that that kind of suffering was good for him, it was

the only way forward. And (as he once told me himself) he was
not a coward. It was more, I mused, as though he felt triumphed
over by my eagerness—as though I were jubilant over his fall,
rather than joyfully nurturing his development. Again I regretted
the fading of the maternal transference, though I assumed it
would be only temporary. I expected him to oscillate on this
threshold for some time, as with our struggle over the Grave.
Instead, he slipped away from me altogether.

The warning signs first appeared when Hamlet recounted to
me his first (inevitable) chance encounter with Ophelia after she
had come out of hospital. It was, of course, what he had been
dreading; but I was convinced that once it had happened, he
would soon assimilate the experience into his life, and it would
prove fruitful in the long run, however uncomfortable at the time.
He began wryly enough and with a tinge of humour:

"I saw her under the arches in the Market. She was standing
by a pillar looking at the rain falling in the square. As soon as she
came round the corner I realized it was her, though she had her
back to me. My head crept right down into my scarf, in fact it's
given me a crick in the neck. You know, that Shakespeare poem
about 'the snail, whose tender horns being hit'—'shelly pain' and
all that. There were loads of people about. I thought I might get
away without her noticing me."

Here he paused and seemed reluctant to continue.

"But I didn't", he said with a note of finality. "She turned
around and saw me."

He said this as though his doom were sealed. I was puzzled at
his making such a drama of it.

"Of course, she was a bit embarrassed. Only for a few seconds.
Then she had a good look at me. I knew she was feeling sorry for
me, because I am such a wreck. And then I realized, with absolute
certainty, that it had to be all over between us. I suppose till then,
I must have secretly imagined we might somehow have picked it
up again. But I just couldn't stand her pitying me, after the way
things used to be."

Is that all? I wondered to myself. We were, of course, back in
the familiar territory of his assuming with "absolute certainty"
that he "knew" Ophelia's feelings, on evidence that ranged from
the slender to the non-existent. This time, however, I suspected it

was not his old tyrannical grandiosity, but an excuse for some-thing else. We could, at least, I said, investigate the sincerity of his own reaction.

"No, no," he insisted earnestly; "this time I really *do* know. There's no need for you to smooth over my failures. I've been thinking about it a lot since it happened, and I feel I can step out now and get on with life. I can face things better now I know where we stand."

Something about this made me ask, when *did* the meeting with Ophelia take place? He replied furtively that it was about ten days ago, and when I asked why he hadn't told me before, he mumbled some feeble excuses about how it "hadn't actually come to his mind in the sessions" and "hadn't seemed that important at the time, it was only thinking over it—" and so on. This particular type of dishonesty had never occurred with Hamlet before, and it made me uneasy. Previous barriers to communication between us had always been of a tangible sort, demonstrably resulting from his omnipotence. This type of non-communication was more like a vacuum. I would have to evolve some new method of bridging it.

However, I was not to be given the chance. A few days after that session, I received a letter from Hamlet, informing me that he had decided to terminate his analysis:

"Dear Dr Horacio,

I am writing to thank you for all you have done to give me some real confidence in myself. You will understand what I mean when I say that now I feel ready at last to face the rat-race of life. Without you I couldn't have done it. You were the only person I could rely on not to play on my sensitivities like a pipe, or to pretend you were suffering with me when really you didn't care.

Above all, I have found the experience of being in analysis to be a wonderful training in self-observation. That, I know, will be an invaluable qualification for the future.

Meanwhile, since we are no longer bound by the psychoanalytic code, I expect you might like to see a few

lines from a long autobiographical poem I am writing, as
a kind of farewell present:

> I don't want to be
> like you, Forte:
> a lapwing running away
> with the shell on its head.
> The expectancy of an MG
> and other childish toys
> won't satisfy me.
> My own ambition is divine, and puffing out,
> makes mouths at the invisible event.
> The yet unknowing world shall see
> my shell will be
> around, above, within me.
> The readiness is all.

Adieu!
with love from Hamlet."

And farewell it was, for the next eight years. Such was my
dismissal by the prince: courteously, the barriers were drawn between his inner self and me. Frequently at first, then intermittently
during all that time, the memory of Hamlet would recur like a
varying dose of miserable bewilderment. I could make no sense of
his departure. Why had he done it? Here again was the lonely only
child; but instead of reaching out, as when I had first met him, he
had chosen to shut himself away, knowingly, in his MG-type shell
of supposed worldly invulnerability, where he would not be prey
to disturbing emotional relationships. After all our work to release
him from a seriously claustrophobic state, his grandiosity had
merely taken another form. And then the unconscious hypocrisy of
it—to pretend to thank *me* for this new pseudo-independence! He
might as well thank me for kicking me in the balls, or stabbing me
in the heart. While I was left unweaponed, with no right to reply.

CHAPTER EIGHT

The King and Queen

KING: In the corrupted currents of this world
Offence's gilded hand may shove by justice,
And oft 'tis seen the wicked prize itself
Buys out the law. But 'tis not so above:
There is no shuffling, there the action lies
In his true nature, and we ourselves compell'd
Even to the teeth and forehead of our faults
To give in evidence.

[III. iii. 57–64]

Despite Hamlet's "farewell" letter, I kept his regular sessions available for two weeks, in case he should suddenly choose to come back. It would be hard for me to say whether I was more hurt or mystified by his sudden departure. It was as though I had been in the process of pulling someone who had fallen overboard back on the ship, when they let go my hand and slowly sank from view. In a variation on Stevie Smith's "not waving but drowning", Hamlet waved goodbye—apparently not

realizing that he was drowning. And I, too, sometimes felt I was drowning in a welter of painful confusion. Had I somehow conspired with him in the delusion that he was "cured", or set on his way as a poet—ready in fact to write his "autobiography?" Had I given the impression that his distress at Ophelia's illness, in both somatic and dream-terms, had earned him some sort of absolution from his sins, which could then be packaged away into the past?

No, I could find nothing in my soul-searching of those weeks to explain Hamlet's sliding away into his "shell", or to match the intensity of my degree of hurt at his complacent and hypocritical letter. I was impatient for information, for new light on the matter. So when I contacted his parents to inform them that he had broken off his analysis (of which, as I suspected, they were not aware) and Gertrude invited me to discuss it with them over dinner at their home, I accepted with very little hesitation. I told myself that what I would normally have considered a breach of technique (given that I had by no means given up hope of his return) was excusable in these peculiar circumstances. Moreover, I found the temptation to see the Danes' new flat irresistible, especially as my own home seemed a particularly cheerless and disturbing place at that moment in time.

It was a fine evening in early summer when I sauntered slowly over the top of the Heath, still alive with strollers and dogwalkers, past the usual gaggle of Saturday-night teenagers congregating round Whitestone Pond. As I walked I meditated on the empty house I'd left behind me in Flask Walk. My daughters were away at pony camp for the weekend, and for the first time my wife had openly gone off with her lover. How was it, I wondered, that I had not seen before now—had refused to see—the extent of our alienation from one another? Beatrice had seemed almost surprised at my concern. Was it some sort of narcissism on my part, that assumed our relationship was invulnerable—was I really perhaps what Hamlet was always calling me, an "old romantic"? Occupied by disturbing and unresolvable musings, I arrived at the Danes' new flat in Redington Road.

Their flat, which Hamlet had complained about as being poky and cramped, was spacious, elegant, and luxuriously appointed. It had been converted with exquisite taste, retaining early nineteenth-century features such as a huge marble fireplace and carefully restored plaster mouldings. These were combined with modern open planning and light. The airy, split-level hexagonal hallway, floored in white marble, had a short flight of wide, open stairs up one side (and a doorway off them, leading presumably to Hamlet's "cupboard" bedroom). All the room doors led off the central hall, including a noble archway to the large parquet-floored Persian-carpeted sitting-cum-dining-room, with a view onto the garden through French windows at the end. I admired on behalf of my wife the stainless steel kitchen range, like a modern Aga, visible through another doorway, and the array of matching pots and pans, all in gleaming stainless steel. The heavy scent of honeysuckle wafted through the open French windows in the gloaming.

An amiable-looking, elderly serving-woman, whom Gertrude addressed affectionately as "Lise, *chérie*", came round with a tray of exotic home-made hors d'oeuvres, while Claude descended to the basement and returned with several dark, dusty bottles of red wine. He set these on the dining table and opened two of them.

"I'm sorry your wife couldn't come, Dr Horacio", said Gertrude, who was wearing a silk blouse and trousers, and jew-elled slippers. She seemed fluttery and anxious. Claude, in a black polo-neck sweater, looked distinguished and genial, with his curly grey hair. For a moment, impressed by their welcome, I almost wondered whether it would be appropriate to mention my own personal troubles. But Claude, with either exquisite manners or extreme tact, rendered any such confession unnecessary:

"It wouldn't have been fair to inflict this post-mortem on her", he said, handing me the Tio Pepe I had asked for, then pouring himself a glass of wine.

No, I thought, I was there in a capacity of courtesy rather than of personal intimacy. Without any further preliminaries, Gertrude asked me directly why Hamlet had stopped his analysis. "It's not because he is—perhaps—all right now without it, is it?" she asked, carefully avoiding the word "cured".

I replied that I did not understand it myself. It had happened when he had just begun to work seriously at it and when I had been feeling most optimistic about our chances of progress. No, I did not think he was "all right" in any other than a superficial sense; in fact, the way he had broken it off made me feel quite worried about him.

"Worried in what sense—you don't think he might do himself some harm, do you?" asked his mother quickly. "It was such a terrible shock when Ophelia slit her wrists—none of us had foreseen anything like that. Poor Antony became an old man overnight."

I reassured her that my anxieties were to do with character development now, not with mental illness.

"It seemed to me", said Claude, "that he had become very much better. You must have done something for him, Dr Horacio. I had quite a pleasant outing with him during the Easter vacation when we went sailing. Almost nostalgic—like old times. As though I were a human being again, even in his eyes."

"But it was evident that he was still very unhappy", said Gertrude. "It wasn't really like old times. He had lost his spirit. He just shut himself in his room, moping."

"Well, it's a good thing he did lose his spirit, in my view", said Claude. "There were times when I could have murdered him. And I suspect he was pretty nasty to Ophelia over the pregnancy business. I think he was depressed because he was feeling guilty— and that can only be a good thing."

"What surprised me was how little he said about Ophelia", said Gertrude. "He knew I'd been to see her, several times. But he never asked me how she was, never even asked about the miscarriage".

"It isn't likely he'd have talked to you about it, in the circumstances, is it—he'd find out from Nando."

"But", continued Gertrude in a puzzled tone, "it was the same with her. She never mentioned Hamlet either. I asked Sister Hertford, and she said the same. It was as though he'd gone out of her life."

I could hardly refrain from expressing my surprise when I heard Gertrude speak of Ophelia's "miscarriage". Clearly Hamlet had not been aware of this—had not had the curiosity to find out. Meanwhile Claude was addressing his wife in a significant and pointed manner:

"I think, myself", he said, "that we were too keen to push them together in the first place. You were, in particular, my dear—you and Antony. It looked like the ideal finale to our family intimacy."

From this point in the conversation I began to find my position in our little triangle extremely uncomfortable. The Danes began by treating me rather like the trusted family lawyer who is privy to the various skeletons in the family cupboard. But for me as Hamlet's analyst (or failed analyst), the situation was far more complicated and uneasy.

Gertrude leaned slightly in my direction with a confidential air and looked at her husband with a sort of provocative, amused defiance, saying:

"Claude's still jealous, you see, Dr Horacio. He's jealous because he believes I had a little affair with Antony once—at a time, I may say, when he was so busy building up his business to be the biggest in Britain that he wasn't really aware of my existence."

"That's a great exaggeration", said Claude, ruffled. "And Antony wasn't the only one I had reason to worry about. But you're not taking my point, Gertrude—which is that Hamlet and Ophelia are only a couple of inexperienced teenagers. Nobody gets married that young these days."

"Nobody said they had to get married!" exclaimed his wife. "There would have been plenty of opportunity for that. And we didn't get married so young ourselves, did we?" she reminded him, somewhat accusingly.

"That was because of the war", he said authoritatively. "I needed to get established first".

He looked at me as if to seek my confirmation, and I was unsure how to respond, finding myself to be an involuntary witness to a private quarrel, yet aware that each of them regarded me as an essential ingredient. Possibly, I felt, my presence even acted as a catalyst.

"Claude's always paid too much attention to being established", said Gertrude to me. "We could have been half as rich and had twice as many children and been twice as happy." She spoke surprisingly sharply, and clearly pained him.

"Are you really saying you haven't been happy with me?" he asked, looking genuinely hurt, his mouth drooping mournfully.

At this Gertrude softened immediately and said "No, no—you know that's not what I mean at all. We've been very happy, more than many people. We've been lucky."

"We've been lucky, I might say, because of working hard", he corrected her. "I wanted to give my son what my father gave me, and more."

"Of course, and you have", she said soothingly. "Nobody could say Hamlet hasn't had every possible opportunity, every advantage. And love. I just mean, perhaps you even worked *too* hard. All those years of you making big money and us entertaining the whole world in our big London mansion—what was it all for?"

"It wasn't the money—you know that", said Claude, irritated that his wife should bring up this commonplace misconception. He began to walk up and down in front of the fireplace, gesticulating with his free hand (the other still holding his glass) in a way that reminded me of Hamlet. "The money was a side-effect. It was the *quality* of the business that interested me. I told my researchers I wanted drugs that were economically viable and effective—drugs that could really be made available. And I always employed the best—and having got them, I wanted to keep them; so I made sure they wanted to stay. My company, Dr Horacio, was regarded as a model of its kind! Gertrude seems to have forgotten all the effort I put in, from the very beginning, towards improving the working conditions. I don't mean only the industrial aspects; I was one of the first to implement the incentives for better morale, which were just experimental at the time—workers' councils, transferable pensions, profit-sharing according to length of service, and so on. I wanted them to understand it was *their* company as much as mine—I knew that efficiency depended on work satisfaction and loyalty to the company. The result was that when I sold out to Universal Pharmaceuticals, my company was an asset in every way. They were lucky to get it!"

He paused for a moment, impressively, and nodded towards me, before adding: "And I never would have sold if Hamlet had taken any interest in it."

Like a mother with a stormy child, Gertrude went up and patted his hand placatingly, while smiling at me apologetically in a way that increased my sense of entrapment. "My dear, nobody is questioning your credibility", she said to her husband. "And if more people were like you these days, the drugs industry would have a different reputation. Yet you say you did it for Hamlet. I suppose that is what I am questioning."

"Ah yes—that *is* the question", assented Claude with a deep sigh, enclosing her hand in his. "It is one I have often asked myself. There, somewhere, I do believe I may be guilty."

There was a lull in the conversation as Lise carried a heavy soup tureen to the table. Claude poured his third glass of wine. It was almost dark outside. I was glad of the chance to digest my sense of astonishment, including that at my own romantic assumption that Hamlet's parents never quarrelled, or at least held no grievances against each other. Then, struck by a thought, I asked whether Hamlet, also, might have had suspicions about the relationship between Polack and his mother. "Oh no", laughed Gertrude quietly, giving me a mischievous glance as she passed by me to close the French doors and curtains. "In all things I am very discreet." She switched on the light over a Lowry painting over the mantelpiece and lit candles at the dinner table. We moved to it and sat down. Claude filled the wine-glasses, and we supped silently for a few minutes, musing to ourselves. Despite Gertrude's assurances, a glimmer of light now illuminated for me Hamlet'ssexually rooted contempt for his parents, which had always battened on his criticism that adults assumed children understood nothing of what was going on. At the same time I was beginning to sense something phoney in the Danes' entire milieu—Claude's "capitalistic socialism" (as Hamlet had called it), Gertrude's cultural entourage of admirers—both of which gave some substance to the origins of Hamlet's paranoia. And behind all this, my ruminations over my own marriage nagged uneasily. Gertrude's accusations about Claude "working too hard" and ignoring her had an uncannily familiar ring. Last night Beatrice had said much the same to me. Had Claude managed to tolerate a situation that I myself found intolerable?

"No, it's something I've thought about a good deal", Claude began again. "Not only recently, either. I first thought about it, Gertrude, when I was wondering about you and Antony all those years ago, and I asked myself if it was my fault."

"No, it was my own impatience at that time", interposed Gertrude in a conciliatory tone, sure of forgiveness, "and—frustration, about myself."

But that was not the track Claude intended to pursue. He continued, almost to himself, and with a certain quiet savagery: "Up till then I always thought, whatever my troubles and difficulties, everything will pay off in the end, because my son will have been launched in life, and wherever I may have gone wrong, he will have the leisure to put it right, because he won't have had the same problems establishing himself that I had. When I consider how my father was almost crippled by poverty in his youth—he had shoes on his feet, for the sake of family appearances, but often went for days together without a decent meal. . . . You understand, Dr Horacio—I'm sure you do—that it's not only material difficulties I'm talking about. Welfare State or not, goodness is a luxury commodity if you are without security. My aim was to provide that sense of security, not only for my own family, but for all my workforce."

I began to see how underneath Claude's socialist ambition (founded as it was on his own fear of poverty, and slurring over the wealth differential between himself and his workforce) there was a veiled attack on his wife for upsetting the family stability with her infidelities. Her queenliness undermined his kingliness. He drained his glass and offered more wine. Gertrude said gently, "Hamlet can learn to be a good man if his father is a good man. That's all he needs. He doesn't need wealth."

"Ah, but that is the heart of the trouble—who is to say that I am a good man?" Claude complained (not without some hint that his wife might be to blame for his spiritual unease). "I have grave doubts about whether I am a good man. I started to have them when it became obvious that my son clearly did not view me as a good man. The first signs appeared when he was about fifteen or so. It was only the occasional snide, sarcastic comment to begin with, slipped in here and there: such as, 'done any respectable drug-pushing today, Dad?' or 'what have you screwed out of the Third World lately in exchange for a few glass pills?' I was irritated, of course, by his self-righteousness and, above all, by his utter ignorance of the complications and frustrations involved. Yet at the same time I could see the grain of truth in his criticisms.

They mirrored the spots in my soul. I knew it was only natural for a teenager to question adult values, and in a way I was proud of him for doing so. I remembered being a terrible aggravation to my father at that age. He used to say he regretted having sacrificed his own comforts all his life for the sake of having me educated, if the only use I could make of books was to fling his faults in his face. Now I suppose my sins are being visited on me."

"No, Claude, you're too harsh on yourself", said Gertrude softly, almost in a whisper. "Those aren't sins. It's natural to have self-doubt. Your father wasn't like you, he was paranoid." But Claude hardly appeared to hear her. He refilled his glass yet again, and between mouthfuls fondled one of the bottles on the table, turning it around. "This is our own, you know", he mumbled, "chateau-bottled."

"It's just a little house on the Garonne", Gertrude whispered aside to me, deprecatingly, "near where my grandparents lived when I was a child." She was trying to mitigate the effect of Claude's ostentation. Indeed, Claude was clearly a little drunk. He began to recollect his son's childhood with a misty-eyed sentiment.

"And yet . . ." he said, "Hamlet was the most delightful child. Till he was nine or ten years old, we were inseparable, he and I. His persistent plea in those days was 'Daddy, can't I come too?'. He used to be fascinated when I took him round the factory— never stopped asking questions! And of course we went sailing together—I used to keep a yacht at Cowes, you know, Dr Horacio. I remember, too, when he was a toddler; he would squeal 'Elephant ride, Daddy! Elephant ride!' He'd never go to bed till I'd given him an elephant ride all round the house, from the attic to the cellar." (This confirmed our associations in the analysis, I thought, with the Ghost Dream in particular.) "Then Gertrude would read him stories", Claude continued. "That was his programme every night. Don't you remember, *ma sourie*, that was how it was?"

Gertrude was smiling now. With a certain triumph, she recounted how she had begun early to cultivate her son's literary tastes. At the age of four, she had read him Roger Lancelyn Green's retellings of classical myths, followed by a children's *Odyssey*, "so that real literature could get into his blood from the beginning". She had done more for Hamlet, she implied, than mere elephant-rides. "I remember", she said, "even when he was in his pram, he wasn't like other babies. He never slept in the pram, he always wanted to lie on his back and gaze outwards at everything that was going on, with his bright piercing eyes—he looked so intelligent! And when old ladies came up and said 'Goo goo, ga ga' to him—the way they do—he'd stare at them as if to say, what are you making those silly noises for? Can't you speak proper English?—and they'd look abashed and creep away."

"We were so proud of him, we never wanted another child", Claude concluded.

"*You* didn't want another . . ."

"Nor you, Gertrude, you must admit . . ."

"Not at first, maybe, but later I did, but then time had gone on, and it seemed too late." She spoke accusingly, distressed.

"Well, we can't always have everything we want", said her husband rather casually, as though following a deliberate policy of not paying too much attention to this irremediable sore spot. "I was the first to be disappointed in him, after all. Yet I always tried to indulge his wishes—caprices, some might call them. When he started at St Paul's, Dr Horacio, I used to send a car to pick up Nando Polack and take them both to school—but after a year or two, was that good enough? No, he had to cycle across London by bike. He dismissed the underground. So I bought him a bike. Not long after that, he stopped calling me 'Dad' and started to call me 'Claude'. Not that I minded that in itself, I knew it was the modern fashion, especially amongst the highbrow arty liberal types he was always rubbing shoulders with. At that period, I felt a bit of a fish out of water, even in my own home. I was working round the clock. When I *was* at home, I saw that people were quite happy to accept my hospitality (and there were always people, God knows!). They enjoyed the good living, company, entertainment they found here—but at the same time they'd turn their noses up at both business and science, which was providing it for them. Via me, that is."

Here Claude paused to drain his glass, which he refilled immediately. I could see Gertrude eyeing him anxiously—wondering, perhaps, whether to intervene. Making an effort, I suggested there was something in the climate of our age that acted against a proper appreciation and respect for science and even medicine. Claude seemed encouraged to find an ally for once:

"Yes, you would have noticed that too, Dr Horacio—my wife never believes me when I say so. But I don't think it would ever have irritated me so much if it hadn't been for Hamlet. I came to think of him as the leader in this conspiracy. Gertrude, you see, would encourage him to put in an appearance at our parties, and he'd come reluctantly at first, but then some one or other of our friends would draw him out, and he'd start entertaining the troops. He was a shy and gawky youth in those days. But he could get excitable in company—and this, I must say, always without touching a drop of alcohol. They all applauded his antics, and I daresay cared not a jot what he was talking about. But *I* cared—because to me, it seemed he was always (beneath the thinnest of disguises) talking about *me* and my despicable mode of life, my hypocritical values, outdated methods, and so forth. You'd think I was the devil incarnate, worthy of nothing but unutterable contempt—a monstrous fascist–racist–sexual pervert and even a miser!"

As he spoke, Claude's voice rose aggressively, spluttering to a crescendo, with traces of the paranoia that Gertrude had attributed to his own father. She had been watching him intently, and seemed to be struggling between her usual tactic of placation, and the urge to rebuff his attack on her hostess-ship. "How could we avoid socializing, with your position and the business?" she demanded. "You can hardly blame Hamlet for that—it was a necessary part of his education."

"The business!" exclaimed Claude. "It was hardly the business—how many were clients of mine? They were *your* clients—clients of your literary salon! To think, Dr Horacio—", he appealed to me again "that Hamlet defected from me for that crowd! Beyond the age of about ten, he never showed any curiosity in the business at all—shouldn't that have been part of his education too?"

"Antony's had difficulties with Hamlet too, you know, lately", said Gertrude, trying to divert his anger. "He said the more he praised Hamlet's work, the more hostile he became, and in fact he's given up supervising him. It's a terrible shame."

"Yes, that sounds about par for the course", said Claude in a jaundiced tone. "I daresay Dr Horacio, also, has found him a bag-ful of trouble. When he's finished with one of us, he starts on another—isn't that the way of it? From my own point of view, things became easier for me once he left for Cambridge and we moved house—and of course, when he started seeing you, Dr Horacio."

He was calmer now and entered his maudlin, mournful mode, the corners of his mouth drooping wearily. "It all went along with my losing interest in the business, you see, Dr Horacio—feeling that I didn't want to carry it into the next era. Things are changing. They always do. Who was it said you can't step into the same river twice, or even once?"

I said I believed it was Heraclitus.

"Well, I had the choice of either putting all my energies into the business or of watching it slip into disorder, stalemate, corruption. I would have been quite happy to kill myself doing the former on behalf of Hamlet, but as he would hardly have appreciated the sacrifice and I couldn't bear the idea of the latter, I chose to retire. Now I just get the odd quip from him about how I seem to be as rich as ever despite not going to work, so how was it I hadn't realized years ago that it wasn't necessary?"

Claude grimaced and set his jaw, pushing his unfinished bowl of soup away from him as Lise came round to collect them and to bring in the main course. Meanwhile Gertrude explained that in fact Claude was almost as busy as ever, because he had taken on an Open University course.

"The pathos is", Claude explained, "I think I probably started even that because of Hamlet. I tried doing English and Drama first, but I could see I'd never be able to have a conversation with him about it without being ridiculed—you can't teach an old dog. So I switched to Law. And, yes, it is interesting. I'm finding it very absorbing. Very absorbing", he repeated gloomily, as he began to eat.

"I think", announced Gertrude after a moment or two, addressing herself directly to me, "the problem is that Claude has always looked on his son in a dynastic light. Like a prince. As if it was a hereditary obligation, or necessity, for Hamlet to follow in his footsteps and take over the business, otherwise the state would collapse and there would be nothing but anarchy. But of course it isn't like that. This is a chemical industry in the late twentieth

century, not a crown in the sixteenth. We live in an age of indi-
vidualism. Each person must choose what they are best fitted to
do. And Hamlet's talents lie elsewhere. It is better to accept that
and allow nature to take its course. After all, Claude, why should
you think your life's work has been wasted just because Hamlet
hasn't taken it up? Isn't the business still playing its part, now that
it's with Universal? Haven't you made a contribution to human-
ity?"

"My dear, you at least have faith in me", said Claude wearily
and resignedly. "Thank you. It's more than I have in myself. What
you say about Hamlet and the business is very true. It is, I think,
something I have gradually been coming to terms with for a long
while. Now if I might be allowed to make an analogous point—",
he said changing his tone, ponderously but with a hint of mischief,
"you'll forgive me, I hope, and won't say it's just petty revenge on
you and Antony."

"Well, what is it?" asked Gertrude, only half smiling.

"I think you, too, have dynastic ambitions in your way."

"Oh?—how is that?"

"Consider. Here you have been arranging a match between
our only son and our—shall we say—oldest friend's only daughter. Now if that isn't dynastic, what is? Especially when the son
and the oldest friend have the same kind of mind—one's just a
retake of the other. Then the girl—the only daughter—is beautiful
like the son's mother (and that has to be said of Ophelia, Dr
Horacio). It's a heady concoction, isn't it—but has anybody considered it might be dangerous?"

"How could it be dangerous? I don't understand you,
Claude", said Gertrude nervously and rather severely. Claude's
speech had become blurred and fuzzy.

"Because the chemistry of their interaction may not be so pre-
dictable", he replied more aggressively. "Immature they may be,
but they have to find their own way forward, even when they are
as obnoxious as Hamlet or as insipid as Ophelia. It isn't up to us to
thrust them together just because we think it looks poetic!"

"Come, Claude, nobody thrust them together", murmured
Gertrude. She frowned and bit her lip, snuffed the candles on the
dinner table and scraped off the excess wax, then relit them. "But
I do see that perhaps we could have seemed too eager on their

behalf, perhaps more than they could cope with", she admitted with an effort. Then, regaining her composure a little, and, catching my eye to enlist my sympathy, she corrected her husband's view of Ophelia:

"And there's much more to Ophelia than meets the eye, Claude. I know her much better than you do. I've always felt a sort of responsibility towards her—no, not because of Antony— because of her not having a mother, and because of my memory of her own mother. She and I were friends, you know, Dr Horacio. It often happens, doesn't it, that motherless girls become either very brazen or very timid. Ophelia has always hidden herself away in her music. And until all this happened, her main aim in life has been to please her father. If Hamlet had turned out like that, Claude, would you have called him insipid?—No, you'd just have felt satisfied that everything was going according to plan. The Polacks needed that sort of *quiet* relationship because they were more vulnerable, without a woman in the family. I can't *express* how often I've wished that Antony had married again, for the children's sake." (These last words were addressed to me, as if I could understand that Antony was another wayward child.)

"Well, I've wished the same myself", said Claude—without, however, any bitterness in his irony. "And what's wrong with a quiet relationship? There's enough trouble in the outside world without having to be treated as a criminal in one's own home. Does a quiet relationship have to be apologized for?"

"Of course not", said Gertrude consolingly, and a little teasingly, "just explained."

* * *

Here Lise entered with the dessert, while Claude shuffled into the kitchen to select some white wine from the fridge. Gertrude and I sat for a moment or two in embarrassed silence. I was painfully conscious of Claude's jealousy. (It reminded me, of course, of my own.) But I was shocked by his desire to humiliate Gertrude, and by her evasiveness. I could see how Hamlet, once his infancy was past, had become a pawn in their separate dynastic ambitions. Indeed, with a struggle, they had come to recognize this, first in each other, then also in themselves. Their intimacy had been undermined by Claude's scramble for money and success, and by Gertrude's queenly salon—evolved competitively when she abandoned her hope of having more children. Now (disillusioned with those years) they were attempting to adjust and repair their relationship, but it was a painful process, fraught with pitfalls. No wonder in this context the coming-together of Hamlet and Ophelia had seemed a "heady concoction". As though through them the older generation could be recreated, saved from the decadence and corruption looming on the horizon—The Great Erotic Hope as a means of rescuing us all from rapacity, stupidity, and greed. I realized that I, too, had fallen prey to this attitude in the analysis; I was guilty of similarly pressurizing Hamlet.

Impelled in some way by Gertrude's embarrassed look of appeal, I confessed something of my sense of analytic failure to the Danes. They had, after all, been very open with me about their own problems. But they seemed rather nonplussed at the depth of my concern. Claude repeated that in his view Hamlet was much better, and Gertrude gazed intensely at me with her liquid brown eyes and said softly and reassuringly that I was "far too modest". I knew they had not really expected much of me or the analysis. Their contact with the profession was a social one, and they had no idea or interest in the traumas or delicate handling it entailed. I was an employee who had done his duty; no blame could attach to me. My apology was just modesty. Indeed, in Gertrude's eyes, it was really a form of homage to her personally, humbling myself before her attractiveness.

By coffee and brandy Claude and Gertrude had become more relaxed and harmonious. I no longer felt I was required to take sides in their fencing match. The triangular tension between us was defused, and I almost felt a temporary inmate of their little circle. Gertrude kissed Lise and sent her to bed. "She's the only one left", she explained. "We used to have lots of staff, but now they've all gone, thank God; we don't need anyone but ourselves. Lise is family. The house is so peaceful."

I asked a question or two about Hamlet's friends, and Gertrude replied that Nando was turning out to be "untrustworthy": "Heaven knows what shifty deals he and that other boy—what's his name, Forte something—concoct between them in the City. His social behaviour is impeccable, of course. But his charm is of a cold type. The English Gentleman is not what he used to be. You complain about your own son, Claude, but you don't realize how lucky you are. And I'm sure he'll settle down eventually, won't he, Dr Horacio?"

Before the evening concluded, however, the conversation returned to the relationship between Hamlet and Ophelia and to Hamlet's play production.

"It was very clever, of course", said Claude, "and I realize that's the modern way, to introduce all sorts of extraneous bits and pieces to liven it up. But to my mind, it wasn't ideal for those two youngsters to be having a type of film-star affair on the stage—that never works, does it. I'm not surprised they split up, quite apart from the pregnancy business."

"Well, I didn't think it *was* so clever", said Gertrude. "It was done for cheap laughs, like so many productions these days. *A Midsummer Night's Dream* is funny enough on its own, without all that jazz and slapstick. In fact, it's *only* funny if left on its own. Hamlet should have known better. I could have smacked him afterwards, he gave me such an insolent look."

"If you're not careful, you'll find Hamlet disappoints your literary ambitions for him, just as he disappointed my industrial ones", warned Claude. Yet again, I found myself acutely aware of his jealousy, and how this was bound up with the feeling that his son had been kidnapped into the camp of the enemy, run by his wife with her literary admirers—leaving him in the position of a mere stepfather. Hamlet's "uncle–father", indeed.

"No, I have confidence in him after all", stated the queen his mother firmly. "He was in a mess, that's why. Have I ever denied he was in a mess? What can you expect after the collapse of his first serious love affair?" (She seemed to ignore temporarily the possibility that the "mess" caused the collapse, rather than vice versa.)

"Tell me, Dr Horacio . . .", Claude suddenly turned to me with a newly inquiring tone. "What is your professional assessment of Hamlet's talents? I mean as a writer, a poet . . . after all, that's what we all really expect him to become. I know what my wife thinks; and myself, I'm not qualified to have any opinion on the matter. It's suddenly struck me: is he genuinely talented, or is he just one of those clever dicks who switch on as soon as they've got an audience?—And then complain that everybody's watching them. What do you think?"

I thought (privately) that in my most pessimistic moments my own worst fears about Hamlet had indeed taken that form. But to counterbalance them I had the evidence of his richly imaginative dream-life; and in my heart's core I "believed" that somewhere there was talent. I explained to his father that from a literary point of view it would be better to ask somebody like Professor Polack, who knew his work. An analyst only sees potentialities.

"Ah, well, we'll just have to wait and see", said Claude.

He offered to drive me home when I confessed that I had come on foot that evening; but I preferred to escape over the now deserted Heath in the cool night air and watery starlight.

CHAPTER NINE

Ophelia at Colonus

OPHELIA: But good my brother,
                Do not as some ungracious pastors do,
                Show me the steep and thorny way to heaven,
                Whiles like a puff'd and reckless libertine
                Himself the primrose path of dalliance treads,
                And recks not his own rede.

                                                              [I. iii. 45–51]

B y now my own newly-recognized loneliness was beginning
to bite. Meeting Hamlet's parents had done nothing to alle-
viate that; in fact, it had exacerbated it. I suspected, though
did not yet understand, that it was bound up in some vaguely
non-analytic way with Hamlet's unconcluded analysis. And I was
still hungry for more information. This was why, when Ophelia
Polack contacted me at the end of term asking for a consultation,
I agreed to see her myself rather than referring her to someone
else. It was not my normal practice, but these circumstances, I told
myself (as with the Danes), were unusual. I almost felt that I

needed to see her: that it was owed to me. And since learning of her miscarriage, a certain ambivalence towards her that I had noticed in myself had been replaced by a revival of curiosity.

As I waited for her to arrive, I realized that the question I really wanted to have answered about Ophelia was, could she possibly be as beautiful as Hamlet had led me to believe? After all, "beauty" in the eyes of a nineteen-year-old boy could well mean no more than fashionability, and I prepared myself to be disappointed. But when I saw Ophelia in the waiting-room, I told myself that she was one of the most beautiful girls I had ever seen. She was dressed in a long ragged-edged green skirt, tight T-shirt, and strange patched and brocaded sleeveless jacket. But she moved with a natural grace the envy of finishing schools, and her face shone out of a Botticelli painting, with a delicate long nose tapering straight between her grey eyes, and bronze–blonde hair half-way down her back.

"Miss Polack?" I nodded, inviting her in to the consulting-room.

"It's all right, please call me Ophelia", she said as she entered and sat down. "I know you've been seeing Hamlet. It was his mother who gave me your address. I asked her, because I need to have some objective advice. My father doesn't know—I can't tell him anything any more, he only worries and gets upset. In hospital there was Paulina, I could talk to her—I expect you know about Paulina? . . . Sister Hertford?"

I saw that Ophelia expected me both to know all about her and to be able to offer her "objective advice". She spoke with more self-assurance than I had expected and slightly hurriedly, as though she believed she had to cram an enormous amount into our limited time. She continued:

"Well, Paulina was the nurse on our ward, and I could tell her things I couldn't tell Gertrude, because she's Hamlet's mother and besides has known me since childhood—she's too involved."

She hesitated, as though these "things" were gathering massively in her mind and all about to demand formulation simultaneously.

"Do you know about my father and me, and Hamlet's family and mine?" she asked, as though there might be a short-cut if she could rely on what I "knew" already. But I asked her, of course, to tell her story in her own words.

"Well, when we were children", she began, "our families were very close. We used to live in the same road, and at first my father lived in the Danes' house; that was when my mother was alive— she and Gertrude had been at the Sorbonne together, and that was why, when my father came over during the war, my parents had the top floor of their house. We only moved to Cambridge when Daddy got the professorship, and even then Nando—that's my brother—stayed at school in London as a boarder. He and Hamlet went to the same school, and Daddy didn't want to move him. You see—our mother died when I was three. You know that, of course. My brother was five. I don't remember her at all, and I don't believe Nando does either, except from photographs and what Daddy has told us. In the photos Daddy is already bald, and much skinnier than he is now. Mother looks very like Nando. And Daddy has always had a sort of reverential attitude to her, almost standing in awe of her memory. He always says it was a miracle, the way she smuggled him across the continent during the war.

"I know other people used to ask him why he didn't marry again. I used to think when I was a girl, that they were ignorant, and it showed how noble and strong-minded Daddy was. He put all his energies into me and Nando—apart from his work, of course, he's always been fanatical about that. You see, he felt he had to be father and mother to us both; it was like a vocation for him, to see that we never missed out. Maybe more like a religion. He has never been religious in any other way, though, of course, he is Jewish; but we aren't, because mother wasn't. Also, he doesn't really feel English himself—I know that. He's taken out British citizenship, and he's a professor of English, but he still feels a foreigner. It's something I almost can't understand, because, of course, I feel English through and through.

"I remember when this first struck me. It was one evening a long time ago, when we still lived in London—the three of us— and we watched a programme on television about the Holocaust. Nando asked Daddy if that was what happened to his relatives— which means, in a way, *our* relatives. At the end Daddy switched off the TV and swivelled his chair to face us (he always sat in this huge, high-backed revolving leather chair—he still does). He said, 'My children, the best inheritance I can ever give you is an English education. This small island leads the world, through its literature, and its ideas of justice and morality.'

Then he swivelled away as if he wanted to hide his face from us. The room was dark with the TV off. Nando got up and stomped out. I remember feeling terribly uncomfortable, because I'd never seen Daddy like that, and I didn't really understand what he was talking about. But later I realized that he had particular expectations of Englishness that were to do with his being a foreigner. And how it was a bit like his attitude to our mother, or the memory of our mother."

Here Ophelia paused and said perhaps she was going off the point. I assured her she wasn't, and she said, "You're not really English either, are you?" I smiled to myself when she said this (remembering the devout English correctness of my grandfather, the rabbi); but I saw that she was introducing herself to me as an alternative version of her father. I wondered what had happened between them and asked her to continue to describe her present relationship with him.

"That's the trouble—it's completely changed", she lamented. "Now it's almost as if I were *his* mother. And it's all Hamlet's fault."

She paused again, a little provocatively, as if to test my reaction and see whether I would take sides on this issue. But when I just grunted questioningly, she continued:

"Ever since Hamlet seemed to turn against him, and went all cold and sarcastic, I've noticed this change in Daddy. You see—it's because of Nando as well. It only became clear to me when I was in hospital, that Daddy finds Nando a disappointment. They're not the same type at all, of course—just not interested in the same things. Nando never even wanted to go to university—he went straight into the city. And Daddy can't bear it when things don't turn out his way. So when Hamlet came along, it was as though he'd found an adopted son, the son he always really wanted—clever and full of ideas, and mad about English literature. They had a fantastic relationship at first. And after a while, when I started going out with Hamlet, I began to feel that it was *me* keeping them together, too. I felt sort of—proud and important. Does that sound stupid and arrogant to you?" she asked anxiously, and then, "terribly babyish, then?"

Again I reassured her.

"It was a bit like the first time I sang a solo with the choir in King's Chapel when I was still at school", she explained.

In what way was it like that? I asked.

"It was partly the glory, of course—knowing I could do it in front of everyone—but it was also that I felt I was doing something for Daddy, because he wanted it. That's a lousy reason, isn't it?"

Not lousy, I said, just not sufficient.

"But then", she continued, "I got pregnant, and everything changed. Before that, I never even asked myself if I liked Hamlet or not. I suppose I was kind of amazed at first that he liked *me*. I did wonder, if it hadn't been for my father, would he ever have noticed me? I knew all about him, of course, because in the first year he was into everything—all the protests, sit-ins, plays and things too. Though he never said a word to me all that year. But mainly I knew about him from Daddy, who was his Director of Studies. Daddy said he was the best student he'd ever had. It was Hamlet who got Daddy to organize the acting workshop on Gawain and the Green Knight, and Daddy decided to do it every year—all in Middle English. I was the lady with the belt in that, because I could play the mandolin. That was when Hamlet noticed me. It was strange, because even though we knew each other from childhood, we pretended we didn't—it was like another existence. Well, *I* pretended, anyway. I thought Hamlet was so incredibly busy being such a big noise, he probably didn't even know who I was."

Possibly, I suggested, she had actually *dis*liked him?

"Oh no, it wasn't that", she said quickly. "I never disliked him, even when I thought he'd gone mad and didn't know what he was saying. I just took it that he was living on a different plane from me. And I had a sort of boyfriend, but that was for safety's sake—after all, I grew up in Cambridge and I knew you had to be some sort of Valkyrie to survive the university meat markets, which is what they call the parties. Daddy was dead keen that I should go to Cambridge. I had a secret wish to go to the Royal Academy in London, but I never told him that. 'Cambridge', he said, 'is Colonus to Athens—the gateway to the heart of English civilization'. So as soon as I knew I'd got in, I became desperate to lose my virginity."

Her tone became harder and a little defiant when she said this, as if testing to see whether I was shocked.

"And I did lose it", she continued, "the summer before going up, with this oafish hippy type at a pop festival in Grantchester meadows. I loathed every second of it, but I was really triumphant afterwards; I thought, I've done it—I've got rid of it! Then I felt kind of *armoured*, and I knew I could face anything, even the University. I did think, 'if Daddy only knew . . .', but of course he had no idea, thank God. Now *you* know, Dr Horacio, and you'll see how horrible I am."

I said she seemed regretful that her first sexual experience had been a cold one.

"Yes, that was it", she said, sounding relieved; "and I know it wasn't like that for my friend Rosalind, for example. Even at school she could always string along crowds of men. I don't mean she was a tease; she just didn't have the same inhibitions as me. It was personality, not looks—I know I'm prettier than she is. Somehow she knew how to organize her life so she only had sex for enjoyment, not for . . ." (she hesitated)—

"Armament"? I repeated, wondering to what extent this was a defence against the impact of her beauty.

"Sort of", she said, confused, "that time, anyway. It was different with Hamlet. There were one or two disasters at the beginning, like the first time there was blood all over the college mattress because it was the middle of my period, but that was just as well, since he didn't have a condom, and the next time he kept fumbling with the wretched thing and said he hated them, but it was really only his vanity that was upset. In fact, all that term I think I was on a kind of a high, I couldn't think about anything else—except sex, and the Play, and him. And I couldn't get over the fact that he'd chosen *me*, rather than Ros or anybody—because Ros fancied him, I could tell. Yes", she said, as if something had become clarified, "I had all those emotions mixed up, at the same time. That's why I couldn't imagine talking to my father or Gertrude about it—you could see the only question at the back of their minds would be, 'Do you love him or don't you?'"

And that, it was evident, she didn't know how to answer, even now. I asked to what extent she believed the Play had confused their relationship?

"Oh—it did, I suppose—it got too glamorous, too exciting, it wasn't quite real. It was like drugs in a way. I can see that now. But perhaps I never would have realized it if it hadn't been for getting pregnant. That, and the miscarriage. Suddenly everything crashed down with a bump. Hamlet seemed to change overnight, I could hardly recognize him. I couldn't even *tell* him; every time I tried it was like banging my head on a brick wall. The way he spoke to me—I almost thought he was *mad*; you know—really psychotic. That was the first time I asked myself, what did I really feel about *him*, as a person—not just about being Hamlet's girlfriend in front of everybody else, or sex and how many marks out of ten it got each time. And I couldn't tell if I hated him or hated myself."

I asked, in what way had she hated herself?

"It was really that I was furious with myself for being such a stupid little fool. The night it happened, I didn't notice he wasn't using a condom till afterwards—" (So, I thought, there was something concrete behind Hamlet's sanctimonious confusion.) "Then he said it was bound to be all right because my period was due in a few days anyway. I couldn't believe it when my period never came. I thought that only happened to ignorant little schoolgirls. I felt cold with fear, because I knew it would have to be aborted. That made me angry too—I thought, why should I let that be done to *my* body, just because of him?"

Here I asked why she "knew the baby would have to be aborted"?

"That was it—I just couldn't imagine having a baby that was mine. Gertrude kept talking about 'the baby'. She tried to persuade me to keep it. And after I'd had that talk with her, I remembered something that happened a long time ago, in that other life, when we lived in London and saw so much of the Danes. I don't know why, but it flashed vividly into my mind.

"It was one winter when there was lots of snow, especially in Hampstead, and it lasted for weeks, which was very unusual. As children we thought it was paradise. I must have been eleven or twelve at the time—it was the year before we moved to Cambridge. And I remember bitterly that Daddy wouldn't let me have a toboggan of my own—he thought it was a waste of money, since we hardly ever got snow like that, and I could easily share Nando's, it was big enough for two—in fact, he thought it was better if Nando did the steering for both of us. So I used to take a tea-tray for the times when Nando wouldn't let me have a go, which was often. Hamlet had his own toboggan, of course, and it was the best type—wooden slats with metal runners. Sometimes Hamlet let me go on his, but mostly he and Nando were obsessed with racing each other down the hill, which meant I couldn't go on either and had to use the tea-tray. Anyway—on the Sunday morning, which looked as if it might be the last before the snow melted—we set off early for the Heath. There was a steep valley at the side of West Heath Lane where we'd been till dark the day before, with hundreds of other people. This time we were the first; the place was empty. Hamlet and Nando started discussing where they were going to run their first race, as usual. I felt fed up and said, 'Can't I have a go, on my own?' and Nando said—as usual—'Just hold on a minute, Phely—you can have a go later'. I knew it was probably the last day, and there was school tomorrow, and suddenly I was filled with absolute fury. I grabbed the strings of the toboggan off him and shrieked at the top of my voice, 'Give it to me, you bugger! I hate you! And I *will* go first!' He was so astonished, he started sniggering; and Hamlet just stared at me as if I was mad.

"What none of us had noticed was that the main run was in a lethal condition, because so many people had been on it the day before and there was no fresh snow; it was worn into steep humps and covered in a sheet of ice. The toboggan bounced from one hump to the next at breakneck speed, and eventually I was thrown off and broke my arm. The toboggan was in splinters. Hamlet went to fetch Daddy, who was furious with Nando. He said he'd be grounded at home for a month with no pocket money. I came back from hospital with my arm in plaster, feeling very virtuous and important, and Nando spent the next week glowering and hissing at me.

"I suppose I remembered that because it was the only other time I'd been in hospital. But it made me feel terrified of the abortion. It was the operation I was scared of, Dr Horacio, not losing the baby. I thought I couldn't go through with it. The next night I woke up lying in a pool of blood. For a minute I thought I was dying. Then I realized, it had miscarried. It should have been the best way out of it all for me: I didn't want the baby and I didn't want the abortion. But it wasn't, it was the beginning of a nightmare. I had terrible dreams; I wandered about not knowing what I was doing. I felt full of guilt, as if I must have somehow caused the miscarriage by having bad thoughts about the baby and not wanting it. At the same time I believed there was something wrong with me and I would never be able to have a child. Or that between us, Hamlet and I had created a monster, and it was a judgement on our lousy relationship. Do you understand what I mean?" she asked with a certain desperation.

Yes, I said, I understood. Possibly her feeling of guilt related also to her description of "getting rid of her virginity", as though she had somehow "got rid of" the baby in the same way.

"That night", she said, "I had a dream where *my mother's coffin was lying across the top of the wardrobe in our old flat in Hampstead, and I knew it was going to slip off and crash unless I could press the right spot on the door, which would stop it—and I couldn't find the right place.*"

So it crashed? I asked, and she confirmed it. It was also, of course, like the toboggan incident, when she had felt bullied by the boys and, at the same time, blamed herself in more complex ways—lack of judgement (not "noticing" the conditions, as with the condom), startling her brother then blaming him, instead of earlier explaining the situation about the toboggans clearly to her father. In the same way she had not told her father she really wanted to go to the Royal Academy, thus depriving him of the chance to help her pursue her own desires, instead of obediently shadowing his.

"But his heart was set on me going to Cambridge!" she exclaimed, astonished. Perhaps, I pointed out, his heart was even more set on *her*. He might have liked to know what she wanted. This might have given him pleasure greater than if she merely fulfilled his own wishes. But she had been so anxious to avoid a battle with him that she had not given him the opportunity.

At this point Ophelia burst into tears. (Probably, I thought, she had never been spoken to so severely in her life. The Professor, I

imagined, could not stand confrontations either.) With some violent sobs of relief, which soon came to an end, she told me that
now she knew why she had slit her wrists. "It was to get away
from him, because I couldn't talk to him. There was no other way I
could tell him I needed to be in hospital. As soon as I got there,
I felt better, immediately—safe and shut away. Paulina helped
about the miscarriage, and so in a funny way did the other girls.
Most of them had anorexia and were younger than me. I could see
they were revolted by the idea of developing sexually, and I
vaguely remembered that as something I had got over, though
I never had anorexia as an illness. For the first time I felt like an
older sister. I felt I had a sort of responsibility to show them a
hopeful example. When Gertrude came to visit me, we didn't talk
about Hamlet, we talked about the other girls, and I got on much
better with her."

Perhaps, I suggested, amongst women both older and younger
than herself, she had managed to re-establish contact with her
own femininity, in terms of being mothered and also of feeling
that she might one day be able to be a mother.

"Yes", she said, "I even felt strong enough to tell my friend
Ros to fuck off when she came in to say I'd only done it to get
him to marry me—and that then I had a breakdown because he
wouldn't. I told her she was jealous of the whole thing—even the
breakdown. Still I hated her afterwards. But it put things in perspective."

In what way? I asked—explaining the humiliation?

"Maybe, I don't know", she said (not really considering this
aspect). "It made me concentrate on what was important—because after she had gone, it came to me that the person I was
really worrying about, more than the girls, was my father."

She was worried about the effect her breakdown had had on
him?

"Even before that. I told you Hamlet was being horrible to
him. And I'd noticed Daddy was kind of down, even while we
were doing the Play—noticed it unconsciously, but I just didn't
think about it, I was so swept up in the Play. In hospital, though, I
thought about it a lot. I don't know why Hamlet turned against
him. But it was obvious to everyone that he had—Gildstein
noticed, and so did other people. He was never actually *rude* to

him, just poisonous and sarcastic in the way only he can be—and all for no reason at all. Of course Daddy turned him over to a new supervisor, but that wasn't the point—the fact is, he was deeply hurt by Hamlet's behaviour. He told me about it just after I came out of hospital—I expect he didn't want to say anything till he thought I was better. He was sitting in his old leather swivel chair in his study, silhouetted against the window at the end—the rest of the room is completely book-lined.

"'My dear child', he began, 'my daughter. Everything I've ever done has been with you in mind—your prosperity and future happiness. Yes. And your brother, of course. It was not simply my duty to your dear mother but my pleasure, as you know. Now you're a grown woman yourself, and you've pulled through a difficult time, I can talk to you a little about myself. Everything Hamlet says about me is true—it's true that I am past my prime, I've been teaching in the same old way for years, and I am stuck in a rut. My reputation will soon start to fade, and the English faculty needs young blood, new stars. But where are they to be found? In the Rosenfelds and Gildsteins of this world? Surely I must be forgiven for hoping that Hamlet, or somebody like Hamlet, would fulfil this role. Who could be in a better position than me to promote him and advance his career? Yet what does he do but stab me in the ribs? The cloud-capp'd towers, the gorgeous palaces, the fashions in literary interpretation—they all fade away, and myself amongst them; I have no illusions of my immortality. But the spirit of literature lives on—must live on.'

"I hope you won't mind my mentioning Hamlet, my dear, now that you've got over him.'" (I noticed that Ophelia's voice trembled slightly when she conveyed this, but she made no comment and continued with her father's lament.) "'I realize that I'm getting old, and susceptible to wish-fulfilment. And that was a bright wish while it lasted—I really believed, and so did the Danes, that you and Hamlet were ideally matched. Don't be unhappy about him—you'll find somebody else to love, you've got your whole life ahead of you. In ten years' time you'll meet unexpectedly somewhere and shake hands and be the best of friends. No, I'm the one who has suffered a permanent wound. My horizons are closing in. What high hopes I had of him at first! I remember— when he came up for interview—his tongue-in-cheek defiance

about the association between our families. He said he applied to
Christ's only because Milton went there and had stayed at St
Paul's for the same reason, not because it was the "family crypt".
He said it with a charming grin, daring me to disbelieve him,
and I thought: we can work together. He genuinely loved Milton.
Another time, when he wrote his essay on "Wordgames and
the Demise of the Image in *Samson Agonistes*"—and it was a very
lively argument, skin-tight to the text, if a bit over the top ideo-
logically—I asked him if he was becoming a structuralist? and he
replied in his satirical way: "A piss on ists—I'd rather have my
balls cut off than be any kind of an ist, I'm not even an anarchist!"
And then he added, looking hard at me, "After all, it was Milton
who said you should never *subscribe slave* to ideologies, wasn't
it?"

"'Yes, Ophelia, I really thought Hamlet was a man after my
own heart. His youthful iconoclasm would be just the right leav-
ening agent for my own wide-ranging scholarship. Do you know,
my dear, they used to call me Spellbinder?"

"And Daddy went on in this way for about two hours, after I
got home from hospital. Almost every day now he says something
along the same lines. It made me feel very strange—both distant
from him, and close to him. I could see, though, that the balance of
our relationship had changed. Now I feel older than him, because
I can see he *is* getting old, and he doesn't enjoy 'the fray' any more
(as he used to call it). Perhaps it was true that he suffered more
from Hamlet's unpredictability than I did. He had expectations of
Hamlet; but I was somehow part of the expectation, caught up in
it. I couldn't see outside it."

I asked if her father talking about Hamlet had helped her to
clarify her own feelings?

"It was strange, because at first I was almost angry that he
talked about Hamlet as if it was so easy for me to 'get over it', and
then the book could be shut for ever. But then I found I was
actually hoping he'd say more about Hamlet and what he was
like in supervisions. It was like when he used to tell us stories
before going to bed. Daddy never read books to us, he always told
stories out of his head, from books he knew so well that they were
part of him. I could match up things he said about Hamlet with
other things in my memory that I somehow never paid attention

to when they happened. As if piecing together a story—I could say, yes, that's what he was like. For example, I remember the time when he was sitting in front of the gas fire in his room and he started laughing and reading a bit out of his book—it was the letters of Keats. He held his pencil up and put his foot on the fender and said, "perhaps that was the position John Keats was sitting in, when he wondered what was the position Shakespeare sat in when he began 'To be or not to be'." He seemed to think that was hilariously funny, I'm not quite sure why (it was to do with what Keats had written about Shakespeare). But in some strange way it seemed to be about *us*, and it made me laugh too—I felt so light-hearted, you know, *happy*."

I pointed out to Ophelia that she said this almost as if it were a revelation that there really was such a thing as "happiness" to be had. She sounded a little taken aback, as though I might be misunderstanding the main import of her speech.

"What I mean is—looking back on it, those were the best times", she explained, "not the Play, or anything. But I can only look back at all because I know it's all over. It's the one thing I can be certain of. Have I got time to tell you one more thing? . . . You know what made me decide to get in touch with you? It was when I bumped into Hamlet for the first time since all this happened. It was in the Market. I saw he was looking miserable, and I wanted to say it was my fault too, but I couldn't. I was afraid he might explode. I still didn't trust his temper. So you see how it is", she said with a note of finality.

And indeed, with frustration, I saw how it was and saw my helplessness to do anything about it. Ophelia had one more question for me before she left:

"Tell me, Dr Horacio—was it really my fault? I'm worried I might be a complete bitch. What do you really think?"

It was not, of course, a question that required an answer. I saw that Ophelia had come to me for absolution, with regard to her mental disturbance after the miscarriage, and also troubled by the effect this had had on her father and to some extent on Hamlet. The act of confession was what she wanted, rather than any more specific aid; and doubtless, had her father not become so dependent on her, she would have confided in him. Probably she had been accustomed to do so throughout her life. And she, at least, had learned from her experience of the past year. Nevertheless I offered, should she wish it, to arrange for her to see someone therapeutically on a regular basis. I explained that I could not see her myself, since I was still hoping that Hamlet would return to his analysis at some point. She never did take up this offer, however, and it was some years before I had news of her again.

After she had gone, as I had a cancellation, I estimated I had time for a brisk walk across the Vale of Health to the soothing lawns of Kenwood House and back. Hamlet's desertion, Ophelia's beauty, and Beatrice's alienation were ringing the changes in my mind, confirming my confusion and vague sense of guilt. Nothing, however, led me to any soothing conclusions, or even to any clarification of thought.

Bottom's Dream

HAMLET: I lov'd Ophelia. Forty thousand brothers
Could not with all their quantity of love
Make up my sum . . .
Woo't weep, woo't fight, woo't fast, woo't tear thyself,
Woo't drink up eisel, eat a crocodile?
I'll do it. Dost come here to whine,
To outface me with leaping in her grave?

[V. i. 264–73]

My further acquaintance with the Danes and Polacks left me with mixed feelings. I was more conscious than ever of the seductiveness of Hamlet's home environment, this nest of sensitive and cultured opportunity in which no expense was spared. Polack, too, in his way, was an agent or offshoot from this. I remembered Hamlet saying, "No one wants a feller with a social disease". Now I was in a position to understand better the social aspects of the disease by which both their houses were plagued—the confusion over status and privilege, the loss of identity, fear of being overwhelmed by a new dark age of cynicism and greed, and guilt at personal failings or past mistakes that may have helped to induce it. This was, to some extent, the spirit of the age, pressing on all of us. But I was disillusioned by the degree to which Claude and Gertrude had fallen prey to it, and I regretted not having given due weight to Hamlet's own adolescent struggle, his fight against it. This was the fault of my own blindness, my idealization of his princely origins.

And now the impact of Ophelia's beauty widened my perspective on the nature of this struggle. Before meeting her myself, I had suspected that her "beauty" was primarily an aspect of Hamlet's own arrogance, a label to make her match his own princely status. I understood now that it was a genuine source of emotional turbulence. I also saw how little Hamlet knew her, how his curiosity had somehow stopped at the barrier of beauty. The grandiosity of her father (not unlike Claude's) now became evident. But Ophelia showed herself to have enough spirited potential to emerge from her meek, flat obedience, while respecting his vulnerability.

Indeed, the meeting with Ophelia remained a romantic glow at the back of my mind, a symbol of hope over the following years. During this period I maintained occasional social contact with the Danes and learned of Ophelia's marriage. This did not affect the idea I had that in some way she represented the key to Hamlet's rejuvenation and the resuscitation of his abortive analysis. My hopes, of course, lay as much in analysis as in marriage, and I had been disappointed that Ophelia had never asked me for a referral. It was eight years before I heard from Hamlet again, and all the while I had been awaiting his return. It was a bad time in my own life. I had gradually come to accept the irretrievable breakdown of my relationship with my wife, although until recently we had still lived together. My daughters were causing me some anxiety, and the bitterness of Beatrice's long-expected departure still stung. In a strange way I seemed to believe that I could not make proper headway with my own problems until I understood the mystery of Hamlet and *his* departure, which had taken such a hold on my mind. Then, in November 1981, I suddenly received a request from Hamlet for an appointment. It was shortly after the death of his father.

I had not seen him during those eight years, but his progress in life was not unknown to me. In fact, I had observed his career with some concern. For the last three or four years he had been writing a regular column for *The Dictator*, that organ of the thinking classes whose large leafy pages I allowed (in common with everybody else) to float freely above and about me on Sunday afternoons in the garden, the lounging chair locking both mind and body in a state of idle stupefaction, which was given a nightmare quality by the strange juxtaposition of images in one's head: female buttocks superimposed on pot-bellied children served up as haute cuisine; sofa beds and gigantic tin-openers slicing brown-skinned youths to pieces in full colour. There was, indeed, a variety of entertainments—something for every bit of the mindlessness. Jumbled into a sickly haze after lunch, the conscience of consumerism rotated grumblingly through one's bowels.

Amidst the haze I could not help noticing, and from time to time glancing through, Hamlet's contributions. They gave me no pleasure, and I never pursued further the longer articles or books that he was doubtless also producing for the industry of the printed word. His was a "serious" column, designed for the conscience side of the mindlessness and flirting occasionally with the cultural side. He wrote on subjects ranging from politics in South America to ecology and the consumerization of conscience. His research seemed impeccable and his conclusions worthy. But it pained me to suspect that his "youthful iconoclasm" (as Professor Polack had termed it) might be merging into step-ahead fashionability; as soon as a topic became fashionable, he dropped it and took up the one in advance. If this was his idiosyncratic view of the status he wished to preserve, it was a far cry from his early passionate interest in literature. Occasionally, also, he printed a poem of his own. This would usually be about the inevitable failure of yet another inadequate and meaningless relationship, written with a certain facile, facetious flair. To my mind, their literary merit seemed negligible, and they even lacked the vitality of the one or two coarse juvenile verses that had come to my attention during his analysis.

Consequently, when he asked to see me again, amongst the mixed emotions that sprung up in me was a revived hope that perhaps he was dissatisfied with his present mode of life.

He seemed pleased to see me when he entered, looking dapper, dark and handsome, and (apart from his slighter build) very much more like his father than formerly, with the same ironic, melancholy mouth and cropped hair that had even become slightly wavy.

"Hail, Dr Horacio, well met after this many a day", he said debonairly, shaking hands but allowing his glance to slip past mine and rove quickly over the room to detect any changes. "Same old carpet", he added in the same artificially jovial tone, and then before lying down he handed me a glossy paperback, saying "My latest book—I bet you haven't read it yet. It's called *Where Are We Now?*"

With distaste I placed this volume on the side-table and waited for him to begin.

"I expect you know, my father died two months ago?"

Yes, I said; I was sorry.

"I was sorry too. I was sorry I'd never really let him into my life again. And now it's too late. When he died, I imagined you telling me I'd treated him badly. I remember his expression when I refused to let him give me the deposit for a house, a couple of years ago. 'Keep the Danegeld, Dad', I said—it was a joke, that's what I used to call my pocket-money. I remember how his face fell. It was the first time I'd called him Dad for years, too."

And now, I said, he regretted his ingratitude.

"You see", said Hamlet defensively, "I thought he'd understand—after all, when he was my age he must have wanted to prove himself too. That's why I never accepted any money from him from the time I left University."

Whereas now, I presumed, he had accepted it all. I wondered whether it was indeed his father's death that was the stimulus for his coming to see me—his feelings of guilt at a relationship that had never been repaired, made worse by the burden of financial inheritance.

"It's true I feel guilty", he admitted, "but I don't give a damn about the money one way or the other. It's the relationship. I've come to see you because I know you're not affected by the sort of hypersensitivities that suspend sound judgement and make people see my motives in the wrong light. Perhaps you'll believe me when I tell you I went to see Professor Polack last week—for the first time since I left Cambridge."

Had Professor Polack regarded him in the "wrong light", then, I asked?

"Not now, no—in fact, he was really pleased to see me. That's the point—I regretted not going before. I suppose I went to make up somehow for not seeing my father more."

Perhaps, I suggested, he had come to see me for the same reason. He rejected this adamantly: "Oh no, Dr Horacio, it's quite different. Not only is Polly physically frail, he's out of touch— even though in some ways his mind's as sharp as a pin. I guess it was good to see him because it made a refreshing change from the real world."

The real world? I queried.

"The pressures of the system—you'll see when you read my book, they're all exposed in it" ("where we are now", I reminded myself). "You'll see how it is that Gildstein's ended up running a pension fund racket, and Rosenfeld manages a firm of trainee consultant managers, and Nando is in Bahrain screwing money out of the Arabs—while Forte, of course, has got a special government commission to sell arms on all sides."

And what about Hamlet himself "now?" I demanded rather testily.

"Well, I reckon I'm coming to the end of the road with *The Dictator*", he announced (at which my spirits brightened). "It was good while it lasted—helped me maintain my independence. I never had to sell my soul for yuppy lucre. But I'm getting sick of it—I've decided I need to change my lifestyle, it's blocking my creativity. On *The Dictator* there's nobody whose main preoccupation isn't whose arse they are going to lick or be licked by next. It's as bad as any parochial rag from that point of view. You remember the abominable Mrs Forte?" (he spoke confidentially, humorously, as if this were a joke we could share); "she got me a job on it in the first place. After Cambridge, you see, I knew I had to get away somewhere really different or I'd die of claustrophobia—I hated my last year there, and I could see academic English was finished. So I told the paper—on impulse—that I wanted to go to Argentina; and I went there, then to Nicaragua, then Chile."

He recounted the year or two he had spent reporting from South America and how he had come to the conclusion it "wasn't really his scene" and decided to concentrate on ecological issues. "Those were on a scale I felt I could do something about. Did you read my investigations of the dioxin disaster at Seveso, and the St Rocher scandal? Those big chemical conglomerates are shit. But I never attacked Universal, because of my father. I knew he'd have taken it personally. Though they're no better than the others. So you see—I did spare some thought for his feelings, even when I had to establish myself."

I recognized that phrase "establish myself" from his father. Hamlet seemed unaware of how his own grandiosity, in its sanctimonious ecological form, paralleled that of his father with his benign "socialist" patriarchy. He had always been vulnerable to patronization (despite his contempt for it), and I blamed myself for the time I had wasted on moral lecturing, which had done nothing but confirm his sanctimony, as appeared now in his journalism.

"But now I need a change of scene", he pointed out. "Now I'm financially independent, I'm thinking of giving up the journalism apart from maybe some freelance stuff and taking a long break in Tuscany so that I can just *write!*"

Of course he had always known that his "independence" would be backed ultimately by the security of his father's money. And it was becoming apparent that his wish to change his lifestyle was not founded on any deep dissatisfaction with himself. My hopes that he wished to resume analysis began to fade. But I needed to know more about his personal relationships, and this indeed seemed to be what he really wanted to talk about. He explained that when in Chile he had met an American woman— "Cis, a journalist"—with whom he had lived on and off for four years. "She was older than me. She had been there ever since the Allende government was toppled by the CIA and the massacres began. Even when I was back here, she was always going to and from South America. She was really committed. I admired her. She still sends me copy, though we haven't been lovers for a long time."

And then, Cis dismissed, he described how Ophelia had re-entered his thoughts after a chance encounter with her on leaving Polack's house in Cambridge after his visit.

"Remember how often I used to accuse you of being a romanticist?" he teased; "well, now you'll say that I am one too."

His rather unctuous tone made me wary. But had we at last got to the reason for his requesting this consultation with me? He described how as he shut the front door, he saw Ophelia get out of her car and usher two small children towards the house. "She's had her hair cut short, and she had her back to me, but I knew immediately it was her. It was like that other time—you remember—in the Market, after she came out of hospital. I could see she looked startled, but she was quite friendly—we said a few things—then . . ." Here Hamlet hesitated awkwardly, before forcing himself to say: "The thing was, when she said goodbye, she touched my hand for a second. I felt as though an electric shock was going through me. It made my hand burn."

He raised his hand slightly and looked at it, as if he half expected the stigma to be visible. I suggested he had been rather bowled over by actually seeing Ophelia again, presumably for the first time since leaving Cambridge, and he agreed. Polack had told him, amongst other things, that Ophelia had not had an abortion but a miscarriage all those years ago ("so, you see, she never actually got rid of my baby, not on purpose") and that she was in the process of getting divorced from her husband. But it was seeing her and being struck anew by her beauty that revived his interest, together with the touch which he took as an invitation to intimacy. "It was then I really regretted how I'd thrown her away", he concluded.

I asked if he thought Polack had engineered this "chance encounter".

"Oh, Polly!" he said wearily, with disdain. "Maybe—who knows, who cares? He's never liked John, of course. My mother didn't either—said he's always been too obsessed with his civil service career to be much of a family man. But Polly knows nothing about women and what they really want—he lives with his head in the clouds. I reckon the only time he ever had an affair was with my mother, years ago—though they'd both deny it, of course—but what did that teach him? Nothing. He just hasn't got it in him. I mean, she's free and available now, but you can see he wouldn't have the energy to go after her."

So his motive in visiting Polack was less to make up for his father, and more to arrange a suitable, safe consort for his mother. It was he who was the engineer. And annoyed, presumably because his mission had failed—this would lead him to denigrate Polack.

"Polly's basically a loner, you see", he continued. "He enjoys his retirement, hidden away from the world. He's got his study and his books and his college dinners—that's his life; he'll never reach out. My mother's not like that. She's as cultured as he is in her way—she reads everything—but for her that is secondary to a relationship. Polly just wouldn't know what a woman wanted from him. If he ever did. He'd never do for her now."

Doubtless, I thought, Polack would not "do". I was conscious of a slight throb of excitement at the thought that Gertrude, rich and beautiful as she was, was indeed "available". And I was aware that this account was Hamlet's way of offering her to me— what, I wondered suspiciously, might he have found out, or Gertrude perhaps hinted, about myself and Beatrice? I rebuked him for assuming it was his duty, now his father was dead, to marry off his mother.

"But don't you see, Dr Horacio", he said eagerly (as though we were now really talking business), "how useless Polly has become. That and my father's death—means it all lands up on my shoulders. Ophelia too—now that I know what I know about her situation, it's obvious Polly won't be able to help her."

He believed Ophelia was unable to handle her divorce? I asked.

"It's the psychological aspects I'm referring to", he explained insinuatingly. "Ophelia suffers from instability. I can tell you (and this is before anything I got from Polly), she used to sleep around indiscriminately, before her marriage to that tedious stick of a civil servant (and that didn't last long). When she was travelling around with her Early Music Consort, they used to swap partners as often as they swopped instruments. Everyone used to joke about it. So now, with those two children as well, she's obviously in a very vulnerable position—prey to anybody who might want to pick her up."

I repeated that with his familiar omnipotence he was treating both his mother and Ophelia as helpless dependants whom it was his duty to accommodate—with trustworthy partners or perhaps, in the case of Ophelia, an analyst. ("Well, somebody has to take responsibility", said Hamlet in an injured tone.) At the back of my mind, however, I found I was indeed wondering whether I could fulfil any of these roles that he figured forth so tantalizingly. My old romantic anxiety and protectiveness were revived. If Hamlet had really not returned with a view to more analysis for himself, would it not in fact be possible for me to take Ophelia in analysis? ... For some moments these temptations revolved in my mind as real possibilities. Only at the next stage did I come to my senses.

For Hamlet now mentioned, almost casually, that he was considering inviting Ophelia to join him in Tuscany. "It would be a good break for her", he suggested. "And financially everything is taken care of. My only problem is to make sure my mother's well settled before I go."

At last it fell into place. He was hoping to shelve the "responsibility" of his mother onto somebody else, so that with a clear conscience and plenty of money he could tempt Ophelia to go off with him. And I was supposed to be an accomplice in this. I recognized now an effect that Hamlet had always tended to have on me. The possibilities he had conjured to my view excited my desire to step in and interfere beyond the bounds of the countertransference. Now this excitement turned to resentment, and anger at my foolishness in falling for his unctuous politic persuasiveness. Here again, I told him, was Hamlet the director of other people—especially the women in his life.

"But why shouldn't Ophelia join me out there?" he complained with mild irritation. "It would be a good place for her—I've got contacts there, someone who runs a music festival, for example ..."

His father's money, I accused him, had endowed him with a new flush of power. Now he was really acting the prince. He believed he could dispose of his mother in some secure, companionable relationship while he scooped off the princess and decamped to the pleasure ground. (I was furious at his crass attempt to enlist my services over Gertrude in this context.)

"I know what you're thinking", said he, obtusely: "you're thinking, how will I cope with maintaining another man's kids, especially given Ophelia's history—isn't that a bit hard on the old ego? Well, I've thought about it, and I know I can do it. I've changed a lot since those days. In fact, I quite like the idea of being a pater familias—we'll have our own as well, of course. You could look on it as a good opportunity for exploring the roles of nature and nurture."

Angrily, I demonstrated how his old grandiosity—hard and intractable—was here simply taking a new soft form. He now saw his role as "doing good"—having jumped onto the moral high ground to disguise his egocentric manipulations. Here was his old familiar sanctimony. It was the same as his journalism, I told him, but applied to intimate relationships instead of social structures. Now that he had inherited his father's kingdom (in which—I stressed again—the decisive feature was the money), he seemed to feel that these antics were justified. Was this the way to repair his relationship with his parents?

"All right", he said, as if deciding to play the card that he was sure would convince me of his sincerity, "there are psychological reasons too. You see, Dr Horacio, I'm quite convinced that if I did take Ophelia to Tuscany, it would release my creativity. I know it's gone under with all this hackwork and the strain of having to earn my living. You must agree it would be a good thing if I got out of this hole."

But this, of course, seemed to me the final straw. Now, I said, he saw his inheritance as absolving him from working for the rest of his life. His phantasy of possessing Ophelia as a sort of magic talisman to "release his creativity" in some idealized poetic retreat was just his old omnipotence in a new guise.

"Have you considered, Dr Horacio", he insisted earnestly, adopting his serious interviewer's tone, "how it would benefit Ophelia to come with me? For her it would mean security—and I don't mean financial—I mean she'd be in no danger of slipping back into her old problems."

By now, his complacency and arrogance were really getting under my skin. What was this, some mutual protection scheme to be imposed on Ophelia, some emotional life-insurance? Could he not see the contempt for her it implied? More than this—I finally demanded—had *he* considered the damage he had himself done his "creativity" when he had prematurely broken off his analysis all those years before? Until he came to terms with that, there was no hope of regaining it.

He seemed surprised that I should look at it in that light and muttered furtively that he'd "never believed in hanging on in squeezed-out situations. . . . I'm a mover, I knew it was time to go."

Well, now—I said—the time had come for him to tell me the truth about why he had run away from me all those years before.

"I didn't run away", he said petulantly. "I knew you'd done what you could for me . . . and I *was* grateful—I wrote and told you, remember?"

Yes, I remembered his nasty letter, I told him: a transparent piece of insincere rhetoric. *I* was the one he felt he had "squeezed out" and cheated. And now he expected absolution from his offence, assurances to the effect that he had neither hurt me nor hurt himself. No, I said, it wasn't good enough; this time I really wanted to know the truth.

"What truth?" he muttered evasively.

The truth about what he didn't tell me at the time he left.

There was a period of silence. He sulked. The emanations from his mounting anxiety filled the room. Then he began:

"There was, I suppose, a dream I didn't tell you. It seemed like no big deal at the time. I knew exactly what you'd say about it, anyway. The funny thing is, it keeps coming back to me. Do you suppose there really is a repetition compulsion? It would be interesting to make that a topic for a piece or even a book, if one could only collect enough material from different people, preferably cutting across class barriers, to get at the archetypal . . ."

No! I interrupted. (I was not to be deflected that easily, and time was running out.) *What was the dream?* I insisted. After some casual, dismissive grunts, he took a deep breath and capitulated.

"*I was in the middle of a dark wood. It seemed both strange and familiar. On one level I knew in the dream that I was in a particular place on the Heath—I could show you the exact spot—where there is a deep hollow with some huge old trees, and in the middle an oak tree, which, my father once told me, was said to be 400 years old. 'There you are, Hamlet' he said—'that tree was a sapling in Shakespeare's day!'*

Beyond the hollow there is quite a wild bit with dense thickets—you'd have to know the way in.

"Anyway—in the dream at first I was playing hide and seek with my friends. It was a child's game, of course, but we were grown up, our actual age—Ros, Gil, Nando, the usual crowd. At the same time it seemed we were in the middle of a jungle; there were strange cries and noises going on all around, in the treetops and thickets. That seemed to be quite natural, too; and I was having fun imitating some of the animal noises so that no one could find me. Then I got fed up because they really didn't seem able to see me, the idiots, and I stepped out from behind the giant oak with my arms outstretched and yelled 'Here I am—Hamlet the Dane!'

"They stopped dead in their tracks and stared at me with utter imbecilic stupefaction. 'O Hamlet!' Nando finally mouthed, 'You've been translated!' They looked as though they'd been transfixed by the Medusa. As soon as they regained the use of their legs they scampered away through the bushes, tripping over the brambles. 'Come back, Nando, you ass-head!' I called, but he only glanced at me again and ran. I decided to wait; I knew they'd be back. I lay down on a heap of leaves and looked up through the branches to the clouds overhead.

> *"The odds are gone, I thought; and gazed instead*
> *At those strange passing forms above, and as*
> *They vied with my fancy I began to feel*
> *Immortal longings in me, past the stuff*
> *Of dreaming. The worm has bitten, the invisible*
> *Worm which means that boys and girls are level*
> *With men no longer. Here am I Hamlet,*
> *Yet cannot hold this visible shape of mine,*
> *Any more than a cloud, when through the leaves*
> *It presses against my branched thoughts, and alters*
> *The shape and texture of my head. The rack dislimns*
> *And makes it indistinct. And now it is*
> *Ophelia, her dazzling canopy*
> *Of hair enfolding me so straight, so close*
> *I cannot move, and bending over me*
> *She whispers I must rouse myself, it's time*
> *To taste a dish for the gods . . ."*

"And then", said Hamlet, dry-mouthed, his words sticking in his throat, *"I realized why she was smiling. The sides of my face were all*

hairy, and I could feel my ears were swollen and enormous. I was a monster—and she was laughing at me for looking such a fool!"

At last! I thought, I have it—the Selected Dream! The selected fact that unites the whole into an intelligible aesthetic pattern.

> Then felt I like some watcher of the skies
> When a new planet swims into his ken.[1]

How the devil had he come to have such a good dream? I was almost envious. Yes—I found myself wishing that had been *my* dream.

Hamlet seemed nonplussed by my enthusiasm—in fact, to find it rather distasteful:

"It was horrible enough at the time", he said sternly, "but it's nothing, is it, in cold daylight?"

At last, I said, it was clear why he had abandoned his analysis. It was clear what emotional commitment he found himself unable to face, "in cold daylight".

"So—what was it I couldn't face?" he reacted sarcastically in his old manner. "It's just another dream about the Mousetrap fiasco—didn't I grovel over that sufficiently to meet your exacting standards?"

It was typical of him to assume the dream was about his humiliation, I said—about making an ass of himself through his directorship of the play. But here, it was the idea of falling in love that made him look a fool in front of his friends. What sort of an ass would abandon their game, their play, for such a vulnerable position—who would lose his "visible shape" for a "dazzling canopy of hair"? Nothing could be more ridiculous. No wonder he had run away from an analysis that led him into such uncomfortable situations, that threatened to undermine his arrogance so severely.

But Hamlet even now did not appear to take in my interpretation. He still could not confront the emotional implications of the dream. Instead, his manner became harder and more contemptuous. It made no difference now in any case, he announced, since all that was in the past, and as for the future, he had "come to a decision" about that.

---

[1] Keats, "On First Looking into Chapman's Homer".

What exactly did he mean by a "decision", I asked coldly, anticipating the answer.

"I'm taking Ophelia with me. As soon as the divorce is through, we'll go."

Had he actually consulted Ophelia on the matter? it suddenly occurred to me.

"You met Ophelia, didn't you", said Hamlet, with just a trace of his old sharp perception. "I'm sure she'd respect your advice."

I was astonished that he could still be trying to engage me as some sort of mediator, or matchmaker, after all I had been saying about his anti-analytic manipulations. Who did he think I was?

"Of course, as regards all that sleeping around she was doing", he persisted, as though convinced that this tack (of enlisting my concern about Ophelia) was his most effective ploy, "I realize now, it was probably there all the time waiting to come out—considering that in a sense she had an abused childhood, being screwed by her brother all those years . . ."

Here I interrupted him, my memory painfully jogged by some unworked-through feature of the analysis. I recalled Hamlet's wild accusation at the height of his Mousetrap mania and repeated the question I had asked him then—what evidence did he have for this assertion?

"Evidence?" he exclaimed cynically. "Why—I've known for years. I told you before. Nando told me himself—when we were in India. And a lot of other things I didn't know. I was very gauche and ignorant then. I remember how surprised I was at first, in fact I didn't credit it at the time—he was always boasting—but later I put two and two together, and the picture fitted. These days, of course, no one would bat an eyelid . . ."

He talked on, but I had ceased to listen. The swine! I was thinking (remembering Ophelia's "virginity")—Nando, the lying bastard! That was precisely the type of idea to have inflamed Hamlet's sanctimonious narcissism: encouraging him to assume that Ophelia was available for rescuing. If only I had had a clearer picture then of Nando's character, I thought, I could surely have rescued Hamlet from his clutches—or, if only Hamlet had been frank with me at that time (but that, of course, was our persistent obstacle . . .). And then again, I found I was taking Nando's treachery personally, as if his desire to wreck Hamlet's relation-ship with Ophelia were directed ultimately at me . . .

And now Hamlet was leaving, speaking some polite phrases, having regained his composed, ex-public-school demeanour. Both of us knew our meeting again would be fruitless.

"Good luck, Dr Horacio", he said, this time looking me in the eye, as if graciously accepting defeat in some sporting event. No, I thought, *I* am the one who has lost this game. I remembered the "blue sky" of his Winter's Tale session. Had I, even then, been over-optimistic? Was his longing for the unattainable blue sky a feature of his claustrophobia, rather than an anticipation of re-lease? The depth of the tragedy, its full enormity, only revealed itself to me now, when I understood that Hamlet was truly lost; my hidden half-conscious hopes for his return had survived, until this meeting extinguished them for ever.

For the last time we shook hands, and I realized mine were trembling. Some horrible truth, or coalescence of truths, was beginning to impinge on my consciousness. I went next-door for a cigarette, at the same time thrusting *Where Are We Now?* to the back of the bookcase. I would never read this banal caricature of what was once the heart of Hamlet's mystery.

Oh, Absalom, Absalom!

Horacio Agonistes

HAMLET: thou hast been
As one, in suff'ring all, that suffers nothing,
A man that Fortune's buffets and rewards
Hast ta'en with equal thanks; and blest are those
Whose blood and judgement are so well commeddled
That they are not a pipe for Fortune's finger
To sound what stop she please.

[III. ii. 65–71]

On Saturday evening, after the meeting with Hamlet, I took my two daughters and their boyfriends to an expensive restaurant in Church Row to celebrate my fiftieth birthday.

Both the boyfriends were eminently unsuitable in my view—though nobody had asked my opinion, so I did not give it. My elder daughter, Antigone, a slender straight-backed girl resembling her mother, has a degree in Oriental Studies and an insatiable wanderlust, which seems closely linked to the transitoriness of her amatory affairs. Her boyfriend of the hour was a well-built but in no other way well-endowed youth whom she had picked up on the A40 when she had stopped to help him change the wheel on his car. He was unemployed but claimed he was seriously thinking of setting up a second-hand car sales business after this affecting incident—at least, that was how Antigone interpreted to the rest of the company his disconnected monosyllabic grunts and grins. My younger daughter Ismene, a sweet-natured girl, still a student, brought with her an unfortunately too-steady partner in the form of a young but wizened philosophy lecturer with restless paranoid eyes, whose capacity for ceaseless gabble would have made Hamlet—by contrast—look like a Zen Buddhist in the silent depths of contemplation. Ismene both idolized and mothered him, and he received both services complacently. As I watched the meaningless torrent of words catapulting from his mouth, swathed in a sleeve of microscopic food particles, I wondered what I had done to deserve this suffering. Yes, I thought, I am a man more sinned against than sinning.

Ever since the meeting with Hamlet, I had been haunted by the wreckage of his youthful promise. Now, as I looked at Antigone and Ismene, it was Ophelia who came to the forefront of my mind, and a picture began to form of her present condition and situation. I could imagine vividly how she was now, eight years after I had last seen her, and the likely problems and complexities of her marriage and divorce. Observing my own daughters in this context, I puzzled over the perversities of the next wave of adolescents. Would they, I wondered, succeed in contracting even the type of conventionally unhappy marriage that Ophelia had made—a marriage that was at least appropriate in terms of class, looks, intelligence? Or was this the example they were studiously avoiding—a marriage that to the casual acquaintance appeared harmonious, though it was a torture chamber within? Certainly nobody could accuse my daughters' liaisons from even appearing well-matched from the outside. That was obvious to anyone—take the waiter, for example (I observed):

"Allow me, sir", he was saying, ironically, as he placed a new tablecloth over the area in front of Wellbuilt, where the latter had spilt a glass of red wine. Solicitously, Ismene wiped the front of

Wizened's jacket where it was splashed with crimson drops. To do him justice, Wizened had never stopped speaking even in the midst of her ministrations. Wellbuilt grunted loudly at Antigone, who interpreted for him:

"Could we have another glass", she said. The waiter produced a new glass from behind his back and polished it, then placed it with a flourish on the mat.

"I mean, a different type of glass", said Antigone.

"It is a wine glass, madam", said the waiter, raising his eyebrows in mockery and speaking in a synthetically wounded tone.

"Could you bring a beer glass, please", she insisted defiantly, staring him in the eye. So a beer glass was brought for Wellbuilt.

Why on earth did I bring them here? I thought. Was this my punishment for marital failure? In fact, Beatrice had only recently left me, to live with her lover of many years' standing; and the girls would be considered grown up by any normal standards. I found myself wondering how they would have behaved if Gertrude had been there. Gradually, my senses shut themselves against the inconsequential clatter going on around me. Wizened and Wellbuilt faded into the dim light of actuality, and instead *I was seated at a small table opposite Gertrude, candle-lit as once many years ago, but this time alone with her, drinking deep from her eyes and enveloped in her attentiveness to our mutual interests and desires.*

"You see, David," she was explaining, "I've always looked on myself as a type of surrogate mother to Ophelia. But it's been difficult, because I've never felt able to allow myself the direct influence that I could have had if she were legitimately my daughter."

"Sometimes that's the best way", I replied, thinking of my lack of influence on my own. But she, of course, interpreted my comment otherwise:

"Ah! you're thinking of Claude and Hamlet", she sighed softly. "The saddest thing is, how similar they really were underneath. They should have been friends. I always hoped they would be, one day—but now it's too late. Have you noticed that Hamlet is even beginning to look a bit like Claude? He did when he was a baby, too, before his hair went straight. No", she said ruminatively, as though this thought had only just occurred to her, "I don't think Claude ever suffered from the delusion that Hamlet wasn't his. That was never part of his dissatisfaction. Hamlet was much more civilized towards him latterly, of course. But it was only

a façade. You could see that in his heart he still regarded his father as a bully of some kind, a dictator. And yet Claude was the gentlest of men! He never punished Hamlet in his life. I was the one who spanked him when he was naughty, when he was little."

Temperamentally, I observed, Hamlet was probably much more like his mother.

"Little and fierce!" she laughed. "But the truth is, David, I know he hasn't been happy, in the deep sense, all these years—and it's time he sorted himself out and found a permanent relationship. There are plenty of women who would have him, but he always seems to lose interest as soon as it gets serious—yet he's not a philanderer, he's just somehow— distractable. He doesn't seem to see the point of committing himself further. I've been worrying that he could become quite misanthropic. But it's Ophelia I really meant to talk about. I know, David, you'll understand what is in my mind: is there any chance, do you think, that they might be brought together again?"

I frowned and shook my head sadly in shame and bitter frustration. I could not find any words to express my despair at what Hamlet had become, and at what Ophelia had become in his eyes. Gertrude gave me a sharp glance and explained,

"You see, I'm not sure she really understands the difficult situation she will be in, with the children—Antony is four, and Miranda is only two."

"She seems to be the one who's initiating it . . ."

"John's not contesting it, he'd find that too degrading—from that point of view it will be straightforward."

"These things are always messy. But there is no point her wasting her life in an unhappy marriage like that."

"John is not a bad man. Just too distant, and—ambitious. He's not unlike Nando in some ways."

"He's not right for Ophelia", I declared unequivocally. "It will be worse later on, when he gets really stuck into his career at the Treasury. It's probably better for them to break it off now."

"So you don't think it would have been better to hold the family together, at least officially, until the children are grown up?"

"When are children ever grown up?" I said despondently. Gertrude looked at me in some surprise. Reproaching myself for having allowed my own filial troubles to surface yet again, I remarked that Ophelia's children were similar in age to herself and Nando when their mother

died. That, agreed Gertrude, was what seemed to worry Ophelia most: repeating their family history of single-parentage.

"And the problem is, both the children are attached to their father", she continued. "In fact, the less they see of him—since he's at work or away more and more—the more hysterical they get about demanding his company. John just couldn't take it. He used to idolize the little boy at first. It was as though he'd duplicated himself and proved his potency to the world. A sort of little-John. But after Miranda was born, he went off Antony as well. Ophelia once said to me he never seemed to think of Miranda as his. And, of course, Antony was being impossible—it was only natural, he was jealous. But John couldn't seem to understand that. He took it as if it was an attack on him. The more tyrannical Antony got, the more cold and distant John became—with all of them."

Ophelia's description, I told Gertrude, suggested a not uncommon narcissistic pattern amongst the type of men who were really big boys and had a limited tolerance of real children, beyond the point where they could be regarded as attributes of themselves. It did, of course, take two to make a marriage fail. I knew that well enough. But John seemed to retreat from the new turbulence aroused in him, rather than seeking help in dealing with it. I did not think the prospects for improvement were good.

"It's interesting you should say that", said Gertrude with a note of sudden understanding. "Because that's how he treated Ophelia, as well, at first. As if he was to be congratulated on having got the prize, won the race in the face of all the competition. She was an attribute of his, too. Did you know"—she asked me pointedly—"that Ophelia went through quite a promiscuous phase, after Hamlet? Not exactly getting her own back, but testing her power over men, as it were."

"It was the humiliation", I said, "of everyone thinking she'd got pregnant to make Hamlet marry her." (How resentful I felt that instead of coming back to me, Ophelia had engaged in that dubious method of self-assertion.)

"Yet even after all that, she got pregnant again!" said Gertrude.

"That was John's way of getting her to marry him."

"Do you think so? It was her choice not to use the pill."

"She'd have decided the pill was invented by men to avoid responsibility for sex", I suggested.

Gertrude laughed, then leaning towards me earnestly she continued: "At that period, you know, David, I did use to worry that she might become a bit hardened towards men. With all that sleeping around—it had a sort of dutiful, mechanical quality. It wasn't even experimentation, exactly."

Yes, I thought, I remembered from long ago that self-defensive aspect of Ophelia, which she herself had been anxious about. But I could detect few traces of this in my present picture of her. She appeared, to my mind, livelier and warmer, despite her worry about the divorce.

"It was having the children that changed her", said Gertrude, as if reading my thoughts. "She opened up a lot once she had the baby to concentrate on. I think she was relieved to find she could have a baby, you see." Gertrude looked at me meaningfully with her deep, expressive dark eyes. I found myself wondering how much older than me she was—possibly six or seven years.

Then we spoke of Ophelia's regret at allowing Hamlet to believe he had made her have an abortion, owing to her vengeful desire for him to feel guilty, to punish him. She had confessed to Gertrude, not so long ago, that if she had discussed things honestly with him, things might have been different between them.

"Hamlet punished himself", said Gertrude sadly. "Perhaps Ophelia was luckier. At the time she seemed to have more to suffer, but she also had a whole world of experiences to wake up to, after hiding away in her music for so long. Like the Sleeping Beauty."

"She does seem to have neglected her music a little", I said.

"Only since Miranda, really", said Gertrude on reflection. "She was very involved before that."

"I don't suppose John gave her much encouragement."

"Not once he'd got her, no. Though he was proud enough of her accomplishments at first—they were part of the prize he had won. She told me once that she had a horror of ending up like Natasha in War and Peace*—singing only until she got the right husband, then having a brood of children and getting fat!"*

Gertrude laughed merrily at this. She herself, I noted inwardly, did not have the type of figure that would ever get fat. She was neat and lithe. I smiled as I considered their opposite, almost complementary, types of beauty.

"Well, she hasn't got the right husband yet", I announced. Immediately I wished I had checked myself. Who was I really talking about? I wondered. Gertrude? Ophelia? Myself? What sort of web had I become enmeshed in?

Noises and vibrations from the outside world were beginning to edge into my dream, though I tried to fend them off. My head spun, and in a sudden nightmare flash I saw Gertrude's figure slipping away from me like Eurydice into the underworld.

"Wait!" I called urgently. "Gertrude, wait—...". But she had returned to the shadows, leaving me more dazed and confused than after the most difficult patient.

* * *

"Daddy, wake up! You're in an absolute *dream*." It was the clear bell-like voice of Ismene. She tapped my arm accusingly. I became aware that the airwaves around my head were delivering messages of an unpleasantly arrhythmic and distorted quality:

"Once the discourse of the Feminine, so long hermetically sealed from history, has been demarginalized from the metabolical signifying practices of imperial phallocentricity, and renegotiates its sociality with and against the cerebrational determinants which have hitherto absented it from the existing cultural repertoire of referential significations, a new trans-hermeneutic validation of its excitingly deviational status could substantially restage its figurations, thereby unmasking the metapsychobiological violence committed on everyday speech . . ."

It was the voice of Wizened. From the persistent glare of his irritable, nervous, and yet pleading eyes in my direction and the shower of vaporous particles wafting down on my plate, I surmised that he was speaking to me.

"What's he saying?" I asked Ismene.

"Oh, Daddy, honestly!" she said reproachfully. "He's asking if you'll write him a reference."

"Oh yes, of course, I suppose so", I agreed hurriedly, feeling guilty about my absence of attention; "why, is he out of a job too?"

"No, Daddy—this is for a *university* post. It's a new lectureship. In Universal Hermeneuticals. It's interdisciplinary. It would suit Stephen brilliantly, it's absolutely his thing."

Yes, I thought, concentrating on averting my eyes from Wizened's gaze, it probably would.

"Oh, ah—", I responded helplessly, knowing, of course, that I was beaten; "why should they take *my* word for it? It isn't my field at all."

"Dad–*dy*!" breathed Ismene firmly, in her no-nonsense tone. "It's your field more than anybody's, surely. Aren't you always saying it's time psychoanalysis forged links, beyond medicine, with the other humanitarian disciplines and consolidated its wider cultural status?"

I wondered whether Wizened-speak could be infectious, and if so was it venereally transmitted or was it in the particles?

"Ye-ah", began Wellbuilt with a stretched-out grunt. I saw, to my surprise, that he was about to venture into speech. (Indeed, once on his own track, it appeared he could be as eloquent as Wizened). "Without me, David, you're losing out. With me, you've got the tax opportunities. Soon as we get our Enterprises off the ground—yours and mine—"

"What?" I exclaimed, stunned.

"You know, our partnership—David and Michael Enterprises, right?" he leered encouragingly. "Tig's idea, right, Tig?"

"You haven't been listening, have you, Daddy", accused Antigone in her turn. "And you agreed it was a good idea. I told Mick you were complaining about VAT on psychoanalysis. He said the way out is to start a joint business with him . . ."

"How on earth does he make that out?" I said, astonished.

It would be purely nominal, of course", explained my daughter. "It would be in *addition* to your practice—and Mick will have his car sales as well, if he gets the site in South End Green . . ."

"That's right, David", confirmed Wellbuilt. "You gotta know how to play the system. We link up, and you can forget VAT. In business these days—every loss is a tax gain. It's the only way to see real money."

A gain for him, a loss for me, I thought. I wondered if Wellbuilt's hefty frame concealed a certain low cunning, but decided against overestimating his intelligence. To avoid further discussion, I signalled for the bill. But before escape could be effected, Wizened insisted on confirming his new-found solidarity with the company, clearly more relaxed and cheerful now that his reference was secured.

"I agree with Mick absolutely", he piped in an eager whine. "We're all partners now. The days of reductionist disciplines are over and the era of postmodern softhumanism has begun." (I noted with relief that the appalling obsequious, hunted look had subsided from his eyes). "After all", he added, squinting at me companionably, "I'm sure you're not a subscriber to the doctrine of *talent*, are you, David?"

It was a wet and windy night when we emerged from the restaurant. We came in single file up the narrow basement passage, myself first. As I reached the top, the wind seized the belt of my raincoat and hitched it over a railing, so I paused and slipped my arm through the railing to disentangle it. At that moment the visionless but solid head of Wellbuilt, mounting from below, hit me in the small of the back. I staggered into a slippery mound of sodden leaves and dog excrement and fell sideways with my arm trapped, giving it an agonizing wrench. I heard the bone crack. Wellbuilt loomed passively above me, swaying in the wind like a towerblock.

"Get out the way you great git!" shouted Antigone as she elbowed him in the stomach and helped me to my feet. She drove me to the Royal Free, with Wellbuilt grunting repentantly (to give him the benefit of the doubt) in the back of the car.

It was the end of Wellbuilt, I imagined, but he probably wouldn't have lasted anyway. They never did. I knew that Wizened would be a much stickier proposition to dislodge. No merely physical catastrophe would serve the purpose. Ismene had been the type of child who was always bringing wounded birds and savaged small mammals into the house. Wizened was one of them. Her somewhat self-idealizing mixture of stubbornness and motherliness could make her pathologically dependable. I wondered yet again whether Beatrice and I had done the right thing in staying together because of the children. How often she had accused me of "working too hard", of "not listening" to her, becoming "impossible to live with", obsessed with "self-aggrandisement". Stung, yet adamant, I had always reacted as though she were jealous of my work—jealous in a personal way. Patiently I used to explain that the work required this intimate emotional involvement—nothing less would do. Even after she had gone, I felt she must have made some mistake. Only now did I seriously ask myself whether I had really neglected her needs. Or was it that my blindness over the breakdown of our marriage had affected the sincerity of my work?

Thoughts increasingly painful and disturbing were being relayed into my consciousness through the painful jolting of my arm in the car. "Old romantic, old romantic"—Hamlet's taunt was again vivid in my mind. I glanced sideways at Antigone, her bright eyes glittering and her small determined jaw tilting slightly upwards as she swerved at speed between the rows of parked cars in the irregular narrow street, with a gap of a hair's-breadth. Her style of driving was alarming if (one trusted) competent. She loved emergencies and had not yet found a vocation that supplied her with enough of them—"Old romantic, old romantic". Antigone was certainly no romantic. But was her obstinate, feminist hardness, which insisted she only come into contact with men of whom she could feel contemptuous, so very different from my own romanticism after all? Was it indeed so different from Hamlet's hard sanctimony?

As I nursed my arm in the casualty waiting-room, I felt for the first time my own romanticism to be in itself a hard shell, defensive, moralistic, idealizing of women. This was not the faith of my father. Was it against this that Hamlet had redounded when he closed himself to me and recoiled into the hard shell of his grandiose Forte consciousness, a prince of modern society? Like his parents, I wanted him to become a prince of the new age: to rescue it from the oncoming rule of the Wizeneds and Wellbuilts who now crowded the floor in all their vulgarity. I had romantic ambitions for him; perhaps I bullied him with my own hopes, heralding him as the chosen one, a repository for my own desires. Was it because of this that when it came to the point, he had been unable to fall in love—to make the leap of faith that Kierkegaard had recognized, and that was required of him by all the forces of development? Had my urgency and importunity weakened him, and is this why he had slipped away, on tiptoe, out of my zone of influence? And was this urgency of mine, in its turn, a substitute for faith in my own marriage? If I had had faith, would I have stayed with Beatrice—was it I who had driven her away?

When I was summoned to the X-ray department, I insisted that Antigone leave me and go home (maintaining that I was sure to spend the night in the hospital). Much as I loved her, I could not tolerate her company for long—a fact that frequently saddened me. She was a hindrance to thought—worse, a hindrance to feeling—and at that hour in the anonymous hospital corridor the pain in my arm acted as a magnet to a host of emergent emotional facts thronging in upon me. Now it was Nando, with his cynical big-brother bragging. It was not Ophelia who had been much affected by this (she seemed to accept it as a matter of course) but Hamlet whom I believed to have been poisoned by it. Before I met Ophelia, I had seen no reason to disbelieve that those two had an incestuous relationship. Hamlet believed it, and through him so did I. Despite my questioning him for "evidence", he must have sensed that that was just a formality. My too-close identification with him was at fault.

But now, thinking it over yet again as I sat at my circular table in the lamplight in the early hours of the morning, with the dog dozing at my feet and a deep quiet outside, I could find no trace of my initial anger at Nando. His bragging was all standard stuff, and it ceased to matter whether it were "true" or not, it was a red herring. Truth lay elsewhere. Indeed, despite her efforts to "get rid of" her virginity, it was clear that Ophelia considered herself a virgin until her first serious relationship, with Hamlet. And I imagined that even now, despite the events that had filled the last eight years, Ophelia might still hanker after the boy who had first brought her out of the "nunnery" and into the world. My anger at Nando was inappropriate. But only now could I see that my pro-tectiveness towards Ophelia was also inappropriate and had been so throughout the analysis. Vividly a phantasy of the night before returned to me. It had struck me with the force of a revelation, as the X-ray machine was moved down towards me and the radi-ographer made a minute adjustment to the position of my arm. I must have groaned aloud, as I remember the radiographer com-menting sympathetically, "It's pretty painful, I expect".

Perhaps—it had just occurred to me—*it was in this very room, some sixteen or so years before, that a fair-haired pubertal girl had sat, with possibly an identical injury, and a broken toboggan into the bar-gain, in her fury and defiance of "the boys" and the prospect of her menarche. I could almost see the anxious bald head of her father hovering beyond the screen.* But it wasn't Nando (any more than Wellbuilt) who had broken my arm; and indeed, he had not broken hers. Her position, like mine, was essentially self-inflicted. Only now, through this parallel, was I able to understand the extent to which

I had lodged my own femininity in this girl on the threshold of womanhood. I had projected onto her that which I should have retained as part of myself. It was an impossible burden for Hamlet to bear. Instead of waiting for him to fall in love, I had tried to *will* him into it—to enact for me my own being-in-love. Had I not always been a little in love with both those women in his life— "always on the side of the women", as he used to accuse me?

This was a crucial factor in my bungling of the counter-transference. My own weakness had devolved upon Hamlet, my own failure to contain the impact of his "romantic" self. I could not forget Hamlet's farewell glance at our last meeting. It seemed the only honest communication of the entire interview. And now I knew why his grandiose attempt to marry me off to his mother had irritated me so much—because it was in a sense a reflection of my own desire, and not only that, a reciprocation of my own faulty method in handling his own relationships. He had not been wrong in his phantasy of who might suit me, just wrong in his omnipotent and condescending view of such a relationship. Over the years of no contact, this vestigial recognition of a fault in the emotional transference between us had rigidified in his mind, so that I had ended up in his eyes in the caricatural form of a marriage broker. He had returned my mistake to me, grotesquely, writ large with hyperbole—but it was my mistake.

"He's no longer the boy you were once in love with", I said to the Ophelia in my mind; *"his egocentricity has closed in."*

"Aren't all men like that?" she said, looking at me intently. I replied, *"No".* The tragedy of Hamlet was that he had *not* changed, he had merely crystallized, fulfilling his predetermined social role. To change requires a leap of faith, abandoning egocentricity to the winds. I had failed to instil this capacity in him because I had failed in it myself. The analysis had left him untouched, because it was no analysis. Like the Prospero of his dreams, I had wanted to shape his internal prosperity for him, egocentrically, self-directed. I had not allowed his story to evolve and followed where it led; I wanted to be his storyteller. Driven by urgency and anxiety and the unmetabolized shadow of my crumbling relationship with Beatrice, to which I had turned a blind eye for so long, I interfered with the psychoanalytic method, I tried to push it onwards. Intolerant of uncertainty, I had allowed my feelings to splurge out,

beyond the boundaries of the analytic context, tainting the receptivity of the transference. "Heaven and earth in the cage of form"—that was the old Chinese poet's definition of a poem. Hamlet's analysis had been no poem. And its failure, I saw now, was more than a mistake: it was a breach of faith, faith in the psychoanalytic method. "If I had had faith, I would have stayed with Regine". Kierkegaard's phrase throbbed insistently, renewing its impact. At last I understood how those words applied to me. If I had had faith I would have stayed with the psychoanalytic method in all its beauty; I would have followed its emotional requirements through the transference and countertransference. My mind would have been alerted to the pitfalls of my pilgrimage. I would not have confusedly and dogmatically strayed beyond those poetic boundaries, whatever the emotional turbulence aroused within them, whatever the distractions imposed from outside them. It wasn't just the dinner with his parents, it wasn't just the meeting with Ophelia—both of which, at the time, I excused as necessary breaches of technique—it was everything, my entire involvement weakened by non-analytic feelings. Not initially, perhaps, but insidiously, as my personal blindness persisted. However vulnerable my personal situation made me, had I stuck to the psychoanalytic method, I would not have found myself trapped in the net of inappropriate relationships—with Claude and Gertrude, with Ophelia—which had undermined Hamlet's trust in my obedience to his childish needs. Crass, vulgar, aggressive those needs may have presented themselves—even ruthless at times—but as his wonderful dreams kept showing me, the heart of mystery was there. And he did develop during the analysis, his dreams drew forth his promise (perhaps this too blinded me to the dangers), but my containment was inadequate. If thou didst ever hold me in thy heart . . . But I refused to be mystified, I withdrew from the path of unknowing. Things standing thus unknown. . . . and those things, perhaps, forever unknown—the man Hamlet might have become. In this trial of psychoanalytic faith I had failed, and I had failed Hamlet—yes *I* did it, a pipe for Fortune's finger. But to know a man well is to know oneself; and in that I am, perhaps, one stage further advanced than I was when I first began to tell this story to the yet unknowing world of my own consciousness.

APPENDIX

Theseus says at the end of *A Midsummer Night's Dream* that when the actors are all dead, none need be blamed. A play or book should speak for itself and need no apology. Nonetheless, as this novel has really been a form of literary appreciation, the following *apologia* may have its uses in terms of highlighting the poetic structure of the play on which it is founded.

What is it to be "faithful" to Shakespeare? This is perhaps a more relevant consideration than the quarrel between "objective" and "subjective" interpretation—when the first is taken to be scholarly but unimaginative and the second to be an excuse for any limited substitution of personal values. If faithfulness is a sincere intention, it must have regard for the meaning contained in the aesthetic form of the play—the "expressiveness" of the art-symbol (as Susanne Langer, 1953, puts it). The play is meaning-ful; and subjective access to this objective reality is dependent on appreciation of the art-form. It follows that faithfulness is never an attempt to be the last word on a subject ("the truth") but an attempt to *be true* to it.

The novel above represents the latest phase in my personal exploration of Shakespeare's *Hamlet*, which has gone on for many years

159

(including my essay "The Undiscovered Country" in Meltzer & Harris Williams, *The Apprehension of Beauty*, 1988). The modern setting and the extension of the characters' personal stories have been done not in a preconceived way to make a particular point, but in order to provide myself with more effective tools for the further exploration of Shakespeare's infinitely fascinating play. (It was also done to amuse myself and in the hope of entertaining my readers!) The same applies to the psychoanalytic vertex of the novel. With the help and supervision of Dr Meltzer, this vertex (which is latent in the play) has been developed as the vehicle through which Shakespeare's characters and emotional dramas have, as it were, *clarified themselves* for me. Moreover, the play has much about the trials and tribulations of being an actor/playwright, and this pivots via the figure of Horatio into the analogous story told here of the learning curve of an individual psychoanalyst in a situation of trial.

In the fourth stanza of Keats's "Ode on a Grecian Urn", there is a famous crux in which it appears that the poet deviates from his direct observation of the Urn in order to describe a "little town" that has no sculpted existence, only an imaginative one. Yet it is this imaginative deviation, this non-academic liberty, which saves the poet's relationship with the work of art and the values it embodies. I would like to take this deviation as a model for the type of literary appreciation I have been trying to emulate with this novel. The apparent liberties taken with Shakespeare's play (more than, say, a production in modern dress, which is really a "translation") have their origin in a need to pursue further the play's implications. With *Hamlet*, perhaps more than any other of Shakespeare's plays, this is particularly appropriate, since it is a play that supersedes its own "mould of form" (III. i. 155); it seems to lie at the hub of his entire *oeuvre*, containing the essence of past dramas and the germ of future ones. This is why I have used references to other plays (in particular *The Tempest* and *The Winter's Tale*) to help illuminate certain movements of the drama that are only microscopically embedded in *Hamlet* itself, but nevertheless essential to bring out.

To begin, then, with a note on Horatio and the psychoanalytic setting, which is perhaps the most important structural "deviation" from the play. It is a deviation, however, that the play itself invites. Who is Horatio, and what is he doing there? Is he a fellow student ("from Wittenberg") or one of the older generation (he remembers

Hamlet's father)? Certainly he is regarded by the play's royal family as of slightly, almost imperceptibly, lower social class ("why should the poor be flatter'd?", III. ii. 59). It is Horatio who first foresees an "eruption" in the state of Denmark (I. i. 72) and then alerts Hamlet to the Ghost "in his mind's eye" (I. ii. 185). It is frequently observed how Shakespeare implies at the end of the play that Horatio has a story that needs to be told (V. ii. 354), and how throughout the play Horatio has served as a foil to Hamlet, an intimate yet powerless companion ("not passion's slave", III. ii. 72). It is not always noticed that Horatio is also employed by the other characters as a sort of measure of dis-interested sanity (by the watchmen at the beginning, I. i. 45; by Claudius to keep watch on first Ophelia then Hamlet, IV. v. 74; V. i. 288). Nobody, of course, really wants *advice* from him, and, in-deed, he has virtually nothing to say. His ironic interjections aimed at calming Hamlet down are used by Hamlet merely to ensure that he has an observer, or listener, at all the key points ("Didst perceive?"—"I did very well note", III. ii. 281–284). Hamlet has a self-conscious attitude to his own "story" (I. v. 107, V. ii. 30), and regards Horatio as a reliable witness. All this pertains to the position held by Dr Horacio as the analyst (and presumably also to some equivalent function of the playwright watching his dream-play unfurl). Horatio experiences, empathically, everything experienced by Hamlet but on a different level of abstraction; he is one who "in suffering all, suffers nothing" (III. ii. 66)—or so Hamlet supposes, in his adolescent egocentricity. All Hamlet's "acting", real and unreal, is undertaken with Horatio at the back of his mind, starting with the moment when Horatio—like Freud's "organ of attention"—first introduces him to the Ghost, the dream-world of his disturbance. The presence of Horatio in the play at the key moments of the Ghost, the Mousetrap, the Graveyard, the Duel, etc., affects the quality of the experience that is conveyed to us as audience. It adds an awareness of potential self-knowledge that is never fully realized, despite the wordplay hovering defensively around it ("to know a man well were to know himself" etc., V. ii. 137).

Without the Horatio dimension, Hamlet would appear less of an adolescent in turmoil and more of a languid yet impulsive aesthete (as indeed he is sometimes portrayed). The romantic (initially Eliza-bethan) concept of the melancholic man fades before the more univer-sally relevant one of youth in conflict, hovering on the verge of the personality development that focuses on the experience of falling in love. As Hazlitt said, "It is *we* who are Hamlet'. The type of "mad-ness" evolved here derives from the conflict, confusion, and turbu-lence associated with Bion's "catastrophic change", that model for all ongoing mental development (Meltzer, 1978). And in the drama of Hamlet's progress (and lack of it), Horatio is a shadowy yet essential figure. It is this overall picture that enables one in the novel to reflect on the problems of the analytic transference between them and the possible nature of Dr Horacio's own private story.

The play falls into two movements and takes place within a dual time-scale. The first movement is the crescendo that leads to the Mousetrap, the closet scene, and the murder of Polonius; the second (when the corruption imagery is overtaken by an insurgence of sea or water imagery) comprises the faltering ebb and flow of Hamlet's endeavours to understand and repair the effects of his violence. His ultimate failure results in his "death" before Fortinbras (the invader of Denmark originally heralded). This symbolizes his giving up the endeavour to become a New Prince who will "set right" the sickness of the times (I. v. 197), and his capitulation to establishment pressures. In effect, Hamlet *becomes Fortinbras.* His intelligence and his passion, which effervesced during the adolescent period when he almost fell in love, are wasted. He becomes one of the usual old-style princes, dressed merely in the new assumptions and jargon of his time, and our interest in him comes to an end. This is his tragedy, and the Ghost's revenge.

The dual time scale derives from our sense that Hamlet in the play exists at two periods of his life—one the full flood of adolescent tur-bulence, the other some years later on (age thirty-ish, as he maintains in the Grave Scene). Somewhere there is a gap, during which the struggle was abandoned (corresponding to an impression many read-ers have that Hamlet actually got to England and spent some time there before returning to Denmark—a demonstration of how Shake-speare's plot in this play is unrealistic and has to be read as dream-sequence.) In terms of dream-language, Hamlet has indeed been "away" somewhere and lost contact with Horatio ("I do not know from what part of the world/ I should be greeted, if not from Lord Hamlet", IV. vi. 4–5). In the novel this hiatus has been translated into the eight years during which Hamlet's story lies unresolved in Horacio's mind, preventing him from fully analysing his own prob-lems.

When we first meet Hamlet, he has just returned from university at Wittenberg to attend the funeral–marriage–coronation of his "uncle–father" and his aunt–mother. The university and the court indicate two areas of existence—the world of peer-group pressures and values, and the world of intimate relationships (family), which, in turn, revivifies the memory of childhood experiences. The peer-group world is represented in the play by Rosencrantz and Guildenstern, Laertes, Fortinbras, and the soldiers at the beginning. Hamlet's excitable, liberal matiness ("good lads", II. ii. 225, "your loves, as mine to you", I. ii. 254) is mixed with dirty wordplay and banter (II. ii. 225ff) and easily clouded by suspicion (a "free visitation"?, II. ii. 275). The price for being The Prince is being an only child. We also catch glimpses throughout the play of Hamlet's earlier relationships with members of his own and of Polonius' family—a Laertes with whom he fought and whom he outgrew intellectually yet "I lov'd you ever" (V. i. 285), a Polonius who shared and tutored his cultural and philosophical interests, an Ophelia who passed unnoticed until she became beautiful, a mother who would like to renew a lost intimacy yet is frightened of his "madness" and shelters behind the men (using Polonius as eavesdropper), able to speak only platitudes. And, in particular, a father who—like Polonius—was once admired and is now despised, to the extent that he has become split into two fathers ("Hyperion to a satyr", I. ii. 140).

The Ghost represents his idealized, heroic father returning in vengeful form to stimulate and belittle the son who is no longer sure what being a prince requires of him. With "martial stalk" (I. i. 69) the Ghost delivers an ambiguous message to his son to take "revenge" yet at the same time to "taint not his mind nor harm his mother" (I. v. 85). This reflects his own ambiguity as one who flaunts sexual possessiveness and at the same time feels cast out ("unhouseld", I. v. 77) by a "fallen" woman (I. v. 47): he is a conqueror of women and a baby whose milk has been curdled (I. v. 69). In the Ghost's speeches there is evidence of both his genuine attachment to his Queen and of a cloud overshadowing the relationship between Hamlet's father and mother. It is Hamlet's inability to deal with the turmoil this arouses in himself that makes him prey to the vengeful aspect of the Ghost as he circles beneath the stage boards chanting "swear" in some primitive spell.

It then becomes apparent in the play that both the troubled "marriage" and the Ghost have come to prominence in Hamlet's mind owing to the new impact of Ophelia, whom he has recently noticed. (Polonius is, as often, correct in his diagnosis, though his insights are ruined by his omnipotent methods for hunting out "where truth is hid", II. ii. 158). There is a pervading feeling that everybody in the Court of Denmark looks to the hoped-for union of Hamlet and Ophelia as a solution to the sickness of the state (and many private "asides" from the King and Queen during the course of the play indicate their underlying depression—Gertrude's "black and grained spots", III. iv. 90, her "sick soul", IV. v. 17; Claudius' "shuffling" and "limed soul", III. iii. 61, 68, "heavy burden", III. i. 54, "superfluous death", IV. v. 96, and his drinking). On the prince's "choice" depends "the sanity and health of this whole state" (I. iii. 21). The marriage is Gertrude's express desire (V. i. 237), and for Claudius it would have deflected Hamlet's attentions and relieved the "hectic in his blood" (IV. iv. 69); Hamlet has his "voice" for the succession (II. ii. 333). It is part of the play's psychological realism that the characters' personal struggles and failures derive in part from a changing social climate, which they feel they no longer have power to influence—indeed, since the reign of Claudius, both Norway and Denmark have been suffering not from the ravages of war but from "th'imposthume of much wealth and peace" (IV. iv. 27). The "lawless resolutes" "shark'd up" by Fortinbras (I. i. 101) comprise a new style of army, perhaps like Brechtian city-gangsters, slick and affluent—a new type of invasion. The older generation are tired and insidiously pressurize Hamlet to repair their own mistakes and metabolize this new dictatorship. The marriage of Hamlet and Ophelia is seen as an essential feature of this "healthy state", Ophelia being the "Rose of May" (IV. v. 157) and Hamlet the "expectancy and rose" of the state (III. i. 154). The basic assumption in this situation corresponds to Bion's (1961) erotic "messianic idea". Everybody wants it, and everybody goes the wrong way to bring it about (in particular through their use of Polonius)—in effect preventing it from happening of its own accord.

Hamlet's view of Ophelia in the play is contaminated by his belief that her sexual armoury is artificially controlled by some interfering internal father-figure, corresponding to a "painted" exterior beauty (hence the rant in the nunnery scene, III. i, and his interjection "Where's your father?"). This is a view that inevitably prevents his real, direct communication with Ophelia. It is, of course, exacerbated by the court's spying and manipulations; but Hamlet is particularly vulnerable to it since it is a view that he has already projected into Ophelia, in the scene when he intrudes into her closet sighing like a madman (II. i. 77ff), just after he has been wound up by the Ghost and decided to adopt an "antic disposition" (the Batman Dream in the novel). According to one early view of manhood, he believes his real heroic father ("Mars", "Jove", "Hyperion")—the one who conquered Fortinbras in single combat—would have conquered Gertrude in a correspondingly dashing manner that he, Hamlet, could never emulate. In this view, womanly beauty is seen as an attribute of the male hero who has possessed it (hence "grace on the brow", "Hyperion's curls", "the front of Jove", etc.)—he is a mountain on whom the woman "hangs" and "feeds" (III. iv. 55). For some reason his mother has rejected ("lost") this model of manhood and opted for the sensual "satyr" Claudius, a degraded, second-rate, second-time father. In fact, Hamlet has himself really grown out of the heroic model, but the superseding one is more confusing. Claudius and Polonius together seem to present him with a tantalising, fraudulent Ophelia whose beauty is really an aggressive weapon and should be locked in a nunnery for the protection of unwary males. If a man should become trapped in this Circe-like house of "bawdry", he will become a "monster" (III. i. 140). These are the "secret parts of Fortune" (II. ii. 235), the home of "bad dreams" (II. ii. 255), the false beauty that reveals the world to be a "pestilent congregation of vapours", a "quintessence of dust" (II. ii. 295ff). "Denmark's a prison" (II. ii. 243). In this claustrophobic view, generated by the Ghost in his "prison house"(I. v. 14), the potential lover feasts like the dead at a type of "convocation of politic worms" (IV. iii. 20), a victim of Polonioid trickery.

This is the phantasy that lies behind Hamlet's engineering of The Mousetrap—a play about a poisoned marriage—ostensibly to "catch the conscience of the King" (II. ii. 601), but really (as the banter with Ophelia shows) to get his revenge on the confusion aroused by the impact of Ophelia. His involvement with Ophelia has reached the stage at which she becomes the focus for all his "philosophy" (which Dr Horacio, in the novel, tries to bring within the psychoanalytic transference). He accuses everyone else of trying to "pluck out the heart of his mystery" (III. ii. 357)—which indeed has a certain truth—but without realising that he himself is both provoking it and perpetrating an analogous activity. Nevertheless he realizes that in a deep sense he "lacks advancement" (as he puns ironically to Rosencrantz and Guildenstern, III. ii. 331), and at this time makes his most urgent pleas to Horatio to help him (III. ii. 56ff).

Hamlet's verbal attack on his mother in the closet scene is an extension of his attack on Ophelia during the performance of the Mousetrap—a type of perverse marriage ceremony in which women "mis-take" their husbands (III. ii. 246). He then blames this on his mother—accusing her of having taken the "rose" from "the forehead of an innocent love" (the image associated with himself and Ophelia) and of "setting a blister there" (the image of venereal disease, III. iv. 42). In the process of "speaking daggers" to her (II. ii. 387) he spears the baby-like Polonius hidden within her "arras" and presents her with a split image of her husband (the "two brothers") such that she eventually says he has "cleft her heart in twain" (III. iv. 158). Yet behind all the verbal violence, which very nearly approaches physical violence (taking the murder of Polonius as a murderous dream of his own), there is always his own sense of inadequacy and humiliation, which began with Ophelia's returning his "remembrances" to him (his "sins", as he calls them) at the beginning of the nunnery scene (suggesting the episode of impotence in the novel). This links with his own lousy love poetry (whose "vile phrase" is criticized by Polonius, II. ii. 115) and his general fear that he is a novice lover unable to match either Hyperion or the satyr. The reappearance of the Ghost in a very different form during the closet scene confirms this impression that Hamlet feels, by contrast, merely a naughty boy rebuked by his father, come to deflect his "bloody" purpose towards "tears" of repentance (III. iv. 130).

And, indeed, Hamlet does learn from the Mousetrap episode. The violent excitement and mania is dissipated and never reappears; instead, his struggle with depression and a sense of futility begins. (In the novel, the figure of Mrs Forte emerges at this point to focus the nightmare qualities of his caricatural mother, and investigate Hamlet's vulnerability to this female version of a vengeful Ghost.) During this delicate period of hibernation, he learns from Ophelia's own depression ("madness") and her "drowning" (translatable into the imagery of pregnancy). He learns from his own "dreams" of the pirate-ship rescue (recounted to Horatio) and of the Gravedigger who (in Horatio's presence) resurrects yet another version of the Ghost in the form of Yorick's skull; here he discovers an actor–father capable of unearthing rubbishy "equivocations" and wordplay, a father more in touch with his own femininity. Hamlet also learns a little from his own warmth in the first fight with Laertes (his leap into Ophelia's grave), struggling with the concept of whether Ophelia has really become "dead" to him. He learns a little, but not enough—he always finds a way of avoiding really confronting the knowledge, incorporating it into his character structure (and Horatio seems particularly helpless at these moments). By the time of his participation in the King's stage-managed duel, Hamlet has given up the struggle to *become himself* and slipped into his socially predetermined role. Hence the artificiality of his public apology in V. ii. 221ff: he has ceased trying to *express himself* and has begun, like Claudius and the whole line of "kings" (pillars of society), cynically to *make speeches*—the speeches that society requires of him. He is ready, in fact, to become Fortinbras.

Shakespeare tells us that any further knowledge to be derived from Hamlet's story must come via Horatio. Horatio "holds Hamlet in his heart" (V. ii. 351)—in him, the spirit of Hamlet is still alive. So where Fortinbras has Hamlet's "dying voice" (V. ii. 361), Horatio has, by contrast, his living one. But this entails telling his own story of "accidental judgements and casual slaughters", of failures and bunglings. Only after it has been told twice over can it constitute a developmental experience.

REFERENCES

Bion, W. (1961). *Experiences in Groups*. London: Tavistock.
Langer, S. (1953). *Feeling and Form*. London: Routledge.
Meltzer, D. (1978). *The Kleinian Development, Part III*. Strathclyde, Perthshire: Clunie Press.
Meltzer, D., & Harris Williams, M. (1988). *The Apprehension of Beauty*. Perthshire: Clunie Press.

INDEX TO DREAMS